OLD, SICK, AND HELPLESS

OLD, SICK, AND HELPLESS
Where Therapy Begins

ROBERT J. KASTENBAUM
THEODORE X. BARBER
SHERYL C. WILSON
BEVERLY L. RYDER
LISA B. HATHAWAY

The Cushing Hospital Series on Aging and Terminal Care

Series Editors: Robert J. Kastenbaum
Theodore X. Barber

BALLINGER PUBLISHING COMPANY
Cambridge, Massachusetts
A Subsidiary of Harper & Row, Publishers, Inc.

International Standard Book Number: 0-88410-717-5

Library of Congress Catalog Card Number 81-3557

Printed in the United States of America

Library of Congress Cataloging in Publication Data

Main entry under title:

Old, sick, and helpless.

  Bibliography: p.
  Includes index.
  1. Aged—Hospital care. 2. Aged—Rehabilitation.
3. Holistic medicine. 4. Gerontology. I. Kastenbaum,
Robert. [DNLM: 1. Aged. 2. Holistic health.
3. Homes for the aged. WT 27.1 044]
RC954.3.043   362.1'98.97   81-3557
ISBN 0-88410-717-5

CONTENTS

OLD, SICK, AND HELPLESS

INTRODUCTION

The end of the line. That was once society's way of looking at the hospital or "pest house." Admission was a function of desperation. Times have changed, of course. What would have been miracles in the days of our grandparents are routine accomplishments at the sophisticated medical center. Although beset by problems both old and new, the contemporary hospital has transcended its dismal past image.

The county "poor farm" or "poor house" was another end of the line. It represented not merely a person's probable last abode but, more oppressively, the end of hope and value. This type of institution has virtually disappeared as such, but there has been no parallel transformation or transcendence. Those of us who survive into the "golden years" all too often experience this characterization more as cruel myth than reality (Gubrium, 1973).

This book comes to you from the end of the line. Unlike the pest house and the poor farm, the situation of being old, poor, and helpless is not one that we can distance from ourselves. It is happening now in your corner of the world as well as ours. Here at Cushing Hospital the situation meets all the reasonable requirements for being at the end of the line:

1. Most of those who live at Cushing Hospital will *die* at Cushing Hospital. In this objective sense, CH (and so many other facilities around the nation) can be regarded as the end.

2. All the people here are *old*, and oldness itself in our society has come to signify a condition bereft of value.

3. It is an *institution*, and institutions in general are seen as places that drain value and confirm failure. Robert Frost once defined home as the place "where, when you have to go there, they have to take you in." Frost may not have defined "home" in these words to everybody's satisfaction, but he has hit the mark in our perception of institutions.

4. It is a *public* facility; therefore, in the minds of many, it is still something of a poor house, socially inferior to private lodgings.

These negative attributions tend to feed on each other and to create self-fulfilling prophecies. The old person may feel ashamed, helpless, and bitter when admitted to a facility that has such threatening significations—a personal orientation that itself can hasten deterioration and repel treatment. Care-givers may also be reluctant to accept positions in such a disvalued facility where both professional and personal rewards seem minimal. And those who make budget decisions may have little impulse to invest in quality care for a clientele that is "out of sight, out of mind." Low fiscal priority is further justified by the assumption that the ill, infirm, and vulnerable aged could not benefit from first-rate care anyhow. A pattern of financial neglect naturally has its impact on staff and clientele (as well as family), thereby reinforcing the negative expectations of all, and so it goes.

Nothing has been said up to this point about Cushing Hospital itself. We have simply summarized some of the major cognitive-affective clusters that attach themselves to any facility of this general type. The unique reality of Cushing Hospital is not perceived directly, but is filtered through stereotyped perceptions such as those mentioned above. This is unfortunate because the stereotypes neglect the considerable strengths of the aged men and women themselves, their families, and the staff. One cannot advance, however, without acknowledging the existence and power of such stereotypes. Therapy does not occur in vacuum or abstraction. It always involves people functioning in a highly particularized situation. The nature of this situation cannot be ignored, especially if it is riddled with negative expectations. In this sense, one does not make an absolute choice between individual and milieu approaches. The uniqueness of each old man and woman requires individual, personal attention—but the milieu must somehow become receptive to such efforts, and this can itself require much effort.

Suppose that we were to design an ideal therapeutic program for the institutionalized aged. What guidelines and criteria would be appropriate? It seems to us that the following considerations are important:

1. It cannot be an *expensive or exotic* program. This sounds like a cold-hearted way to begin. The fact is, however, that there is increasing cost-containment pressure in the health field, with geriatrics a prime target (Hudson, 1978). Yes, it would be worthwhile and encouraging to demonstrate that certain therapeutic programs can be of decided benefit to the aged. But it would be naive to expect that such demonstrations would lead automatically to the services becoming available to all who need them. If the program looks costly, forget it! Just the fact that a program looks expensive is enough to make it a candidate for oblivion today. One might assemble evidence to indicate that the timely investment in effective therapy will result in an overall cost benefit, as well as the primary benefit in human well-being. Budget decisions, however, are often made on grounds of narrow expediency where the comprehensive, long-term cost is seen as less relevant than the question of who picks up what bill right now. We would rather not have to mention the financial criterion, but the day is long past (if ever there was such a day) when therapeutic programs can be devised and applied without attention to that nefarious cliche, "the bottom line." If sufficiently imaginative, one can envision a time when the bottom line will be human dignity and well-being. In the meantime, we must get on with what can be accomplished in the world in which we live.

2. The program must take into account the *multiple* sources of impairment and distress in the lives of the aged men and women who become institutionalized. Physical, psychological, and social problems abound. Many of these problems are firmly rooted in consensual reality. It is difficult, at times virtually impossible, to select a single target problem and apply a specific treatment. Those who would be therapeutic must somehow cope with an array of problems varying greatly (and therefore requiring a spectrum of expertise), and problems that interact in unique ways that seem to defy generalization. Narrow treatment models are out of place even though, out of anxiety or ignorance, one might be tempted to rely upon them. In-

stead, there is the challenge of approaching each person with a keen sense of their individuality and the individuality of the situation.

3. Time's arrow is *pointing toward terminus*. Younger clients may have severe problems, but one can project a possible future in which these difficulties will be transcended. The aphorism "Time heals all wounds" was not meant for the ninety-year-old woman with a heart problem and kidney failure whose daughter has just died, and who does not have a living soul left to affirm and support her own life. If time is the friend of therapy for the young, it is seen more often as the enemy for the aged. The philosophy and practice of a therapeutic program for the aged cannot feign ignorance of time's arrow. The therapists themselves must have the ability to bring all they can to the person right now, even though the best of their efforts might not add another hour to that person's life. One of the core reasons for the reluctance of conventional therapists to work with the aged has been this unwillingness to "invest" one's valued time in a person who will not live long enough for the investment to show an acceptable "return" (Kastenbaum, 1963).

4. There must be a *philosophy of care*. Presumably, there is always a philosophy of care, no matter what the client population or the specific approach. In practice, however, therapy is sometimes technique-oriented. The therapist is a technician who "does this when the client does that." The therapist or technician works in the interests of the client, and may do so with considerable warmth and sensitivity. Occasionally another dimension enters: What is the point? What are the real values here? What *should* be the goals of therapy? The therapist's personal belief system may be challenged and require deep examination. This examination may extend to the therapist's relationship to the universe. "What I think I should be doing with this client depends as much upon what I think the universe is really about as it does upon specific theory and technique." These are occasional encounters for many therapists and can be experienced as quite significant. For the therapist working with the frail and infirm aged, the philosophical questions are never absent. One can hardly get through a day without drawing upon a philosophy of care that, in turn, flows from a general philosophy of life. It is not an indulgence for the geriatric therapist to be philosophical; it is a necessity.

5. The therapists must be *resourceful.* Again, this is a reasonable criterion for any type of therapist. It is an especially salient criterion for therapy with the aged. One must be able to shift levels of interaction. During the course of therapy one might be called upon variously to be companion, advocate, nurse, parent, child, teacher, student, and minister—all of this in addition to being a therapist per se with a variety of techniques to suit the occasion. This type of therapy cannot be performed on one string; the therapist needs not only more than one string on the bow but more than one bow. The therapist, in fact, must be his or her own most resourceful instrument and must keep this instrument well tuned.

This list by no means exhausts the guidelines and criteria that might be specified for a successful therapeutic program with the institutionalized aged. It does convey, however, part of the general frame of reference within which the program described in this book had its origins. How this program developed, and how it meets or fails to meet these specifications will become more obvious as we go along. Our basic aim has been to protect and enhance the well-being of men and women who have lost much of what was dear to them, and for whom everything that is remaining is in peril. The term *holistic therapy* seems to us the best approximation for this program. It conveys the sense of the integrity of the individual within both the immediate situation and within the context of a lifetime. The therapist brings everything possible to the core being of the client. Therapy can involve many specific problems and techniques but the emphasis remains on the core person and his or her connections to the universe. The therapist, in other words, functions as a complete person (rather than a dispenser of various techniques) in an attempt to form an intimate and beneficial relationship with another person who, despite all manner of loss and impairment, is also a complete person.

Inevitably, this book places the holistic therapy program in the foreground. It should be understood, however, that this program represents only one facet of the care spectrum offered by Cushing Hospital. More will be said in a later section about the relationship of the holistic therapy program to the hospital in general. For now it is enough to state that such a program has proven viable at Cushing Hospital only because a context of competence, compassion, and dedication already existed.

The aged person in the institution is the most direct focus of this book. Obviously, holistic therapy is not limited to this setting; in fact, it may prove even more valuable in other contexts. If we appear single-minded here in concentrating on holistic therapy with the institutionalized aged, it is simply because we are sharing the work we do here.

The plan of the book? We begin with an examination of therapeutic philosophies and modes from the past that are connected to the present effort. This critical survey of caring and healing through the centuries is indispensable for context. A brief chapter then sets the stage for the holistic therapy program by summarizing the situation both locally and nationally prior to its inception. The heart of the book follows, presenting detailed case histories. The remaining chapters analyze the holistic therapy process and outcome from several perspectives and also discuss the integration of this program within the hospital. Before closing, we explore implications of this approach for care of the aged. Our intention is to share, inform, and, if possible, stimulate, rather than persuade.

REFERENCES

Gubrium, J.F. *The myth of the golden years.* Springfield, Ill.: Charles C. Thomas, 1973.

Hudson, R.B. The "graying" of the federal budget and its consequences for old-age policy. *The Gerontologist*, 1978, *18*, 428–440.

Kastenbaum, R. The reluctant therapist. *Geriatrics*, 1963, *18*, 296–301.

1 MEDICINE, SUGGESTIVE THERAPY, AND HEALING

Holistic therapy with geriatric patients is rooted in a long tradition. It might be more accurate to say that it is rooted in several traditions that have intertwined in various ways over the centuries. In developing the holistic therapy program, we drew insights from the past as well as from current developments. This chapter examines selected aspects of the "usable past." The carrying-forward of these traditions to problems confronting us today is described in the chapters that follow.

Two major themes claim our attention: (1) throughout the ages, the sick have been helped to recover through the efforts of medical practitioners, but healing has also been accomplished by suggestive therapists and by healers with religious, spiritual, or psychic orientations; (2) these approaches all help primarily by assisting the individual's own self-healing processes.

First we will briefly review the interlocking histories of *medicine, suggestive therapy*, and *healing*. Next, we will summarize data showing how the body heals itself, followed by a review of recent findings that add to our knowledge of how the processes of self-healing are affected by the person's own thoughts, feelings, and emotions—as well as by interpersonal love and caring. Finally, we will examine the strengths and weaknesses of modern medicine, suggestive therapy, and lay healing. We will suggest that the best features of each approach should be used in selecting and training future healers or therapists.

A HISTORICAL VIEW

Since almost all medications until recently were placebos, the history of medical treatment can be characterized largely as the history of the placebo (suggestive) effect" (Shapiro, 1971, p. 442).

This compelling statement by a physician and medical historian deserves our close attention. An important fact is often overlooked: there were no effective drugs to destroy pathogenic bacteria until the sulfonamides became available in the 1940s. If people recovered from bacterial attacks from Year One to the 1940s, they did so without the benefit of potent drugs. The arsenal of effective drugs increased in the 1950s as antibiotics such as penicillin, aureomycin, and streptomycin began to be used widely. Prior to this time, there were few medicaments available that were more than placebos. This little-known or well-forgotten fact encompasses more than the area of anti-bacterial agents. Only a handful of drugs in the pre–1940 pharmacopeia were anything but placebos. The exceptions included acetylsalicylic acid (aspirin), digitalis, and rauwolfia. A few additional additional drugs could be added, and there might be some others whose actual effects (pharmacological or placebo) are not yet fully established. In general, however, as Shapiro (1971) has noted, a tremendous variety of organic and inorganic substances have been used as drugs, including crocodile dung, spermatic fluid of frogs, human perspiration, earthworms, feathers, hair, the oil of ants, and blood from every virtually every animal.

The historical documents available to us yield the impression that these dubious ministrations, these fantastical placebos, often did help the sick to recover. At times they even seemed to have dramatic effects. How could this be? There are many factors involved; we will begin with a few.

A person who is ill often is apprehensive and anxious as well. He or she may not know the nature or outcome of his or her condition. Fears grow and multiply: "Will I become debilitated? Will I suffer? Will I be unable to carry out my responsibilities? Will I lose what I desire and cherish in life? Will this illness be my death?" Continual tension and apprehension is likely to hinder the self-healing process; in fact, agitated and dysphoric states tend to make things worse.

This negative situation can be ameliorated through "diagnosis." There are many ways to define this term. It seems to us, however, that throughout history, diagnosis typically has meant telling patients what's wrong with them in a convincing way. Generalized anxiety is dissipated by the convincing diagnosis: one has a name for the affliction, and naming the devil is one way to seize control. This promising beginning is then followed by some kind of treatment. We will limit our attention here to treatments of the drug type. The sufferer is given a preparation that the healer, the patient, or both believe will restore health. The "diagnosis" may be wildly inaccurate. The "treatment" may have no relevant physiological effects. Nevertheless, these two steps can help reduce the patient's fears and apprehensions and, consequently, energize the self-healing process. This, very schematically, is the treatment model that resides at the core of much quasi-medical healing over the centuries.

Medical and nonmedical healers alike throughout the ages have boosted the patient's self-healing processes by convincing him that he will be all right (Frank, 1961, 1978). In addition to removing fear and apprehension, healers of all types have reduced the sense of helplessness and hopelessness, decreased feelings of loneliness and abandonment, and minimized guilt, envy, resentment, hostility, and other negative affects. As Frank (1961) has documented, these effects were achieved primarily through the techniques of *suggestion, encouragement, attention, emotional arousal*, and *confident* application of treatment.

HOW THE ANCIENTS HEALED

We will now present highlights in the history of healing, beginning with ancient Egypt where priest and physician were one and the same. These priest–physicians were advanced in many ways. They were skilled surgeons and had even developed specialties (Atkinson, 1956). In addition, the *laying-on-of-hands* was an integral part of their armamentarium. The Egyptian priest–physicians also utilized *temples of sleep* in the names of the gods Isis and Serapis (in a manner similar to the cult of Aesculapius in ancient Greece, described below). The healers offered special prayers, together with their collection of pills, potions, poultices, suppositories, plasters, charms, and amulets. This entire formidable "spectrum" approach generated a powerful placebo or suggestion effect. In the face of this show of concern and expertise, the patient found it easier to believe that all would be well, and therefore could let go of fear, apprehension, hopelessness, and helplessness.

The ancient Babylonians also employed similar suggestive remedies. They added a new and useful procedure, according to Herodotus. The sick were taken to the center of the city. Other citizens who had recovered from the same ailments thronged to the scene. Their purpose was to give suggestions and advice on how to recover. Ancient Hebrew medicine emphasized harmony with God and nature—and plenty of suggestion. The sick were urged to pray, fast, and observe the moral laws most strictly.

In ancient Greek medicine the principle was well accepted that bodily functions are influenced by mental states. Hippocrates saw the physician as aiding natural processes by prescribing rest and relaxation, thermic baths, selected diets, purgation, emesis, and a few carefully chosen drugs (Guthrie, Underwood, Thomson, & Richardson, 1977). The most potent suggestive treatment in ancient Greece, however, was found in the temples of Aesculapius. The healing cult of Aesculapius was widespread in ancient Greece and survived through Rome and into the Middle Ages. The Aesculapians constructed impressive temples that were devoted to treatment of the sick. All the many forms of treatment provided at these temples converged to convey the potent message that the patient would be healed and, therefore, there was no reason to remain anxious or fearful.

This healing suggestion was conveyed implicitly by the total treatment process (Caton, 1900; Edelstein & Edelstein, 1945; MacHovec, 1975, 1979). The following steps can be distinguished:

1. Prior to their illnesses, the patients had already heard about the marvelous cures to be obtained at the temples of Aesculapius. A latent expectancy already existed.

2. When people did become ill, they were told again of the temples' curing powers—a reinforcement of expectancy.

3. The expectancy of being healed continued to grow through the process of making the decision, preparing for the journey, and

then actually traveling over a substantial distance. This pattern of increasing involvement in one's eventual healing can be seen as a significant component of the treatment itself.

4. On arrival they found an impressive site and were shown solicitude and compassion by the priest–physician who interviewed them and took their medical histories.

5. The patients had tasks to perform themselves: for example, praying, exercising, and ritualized bathing in water with reputed healing properties. Among other effects, this helped to transform the passivity of the sick person into the activity of the healer—in this case, the self-healer.

6. "Official treatment" was provided in the form of soothing rhythmic massage, special ointments, and diets.

7. All the patients at the temple supported each other, providing an interpersonal climate conducive to recovery.

8. The total environment was given to a calm, restful atmosphere with soft music playing and soothing breezes flowing between the temple columns.

The elements or phases listed above had multiple effects favorable to recovery. These include distracting the patients from their symptoms, maintaining their sense of worth and acceptance, reducing fears, and inducing relaxation and peace of mind. Other potent suggestive factors were also present at the temples of Aesculapius. The patients received strong implicit suggestions that they would be helped because of the hundreds of testimonials of previous cures written on the temple walls. These were, in effect, therapeutic graffiti. Furthermore, the patients were expected to dream of a God either healing them directly or advising them on how they would be healed (incubation). The priest–physician would also come at night and give suggestions to the patient. At times the priest–physician would also bring along the temple dogs and the sacred snakes. The trained and sanctified dogs would lick the patient's body, especially in areas that were inflamed or painful. These same areas would also be treated by the sacred snakes who were trained to place their cold bodies on the patient. All manners of ailment were treated by these suggestive procedures—pains, arthritic disorders, viral and bacterial diseases, neurotic and hysterical disorders, insomnia, and so on.

In evaluating the effect of various treatments, we must take into account the fact that most illnesses are self-limiting (heal themselves even if no therapies are applied). Documentation now available from the temples of Aesculapius indicate that the large number of suggestive elements in the total therapy plan were helpful in *hastening* the patient's recovery. One need not claim that "incurable" conditions were cured or, at the opposite extreme, that the treatment had no effects at all. The most appropriate conclusion is that the patient's own self-healing processes were facilitated by relaxation, hopefulness, and the abolition of fears.

When Rome ruled the world, the medical arts were advanced in many ways. Skillful surgery was available for such conditions as hernia, cataracts, and removal of bladder stones. The basic principles of Roman medicine, however (as expounded by Galen), agreed with those of Hippocrates and the ancient Greeks. The physician's role was to *assist nature* by prescribing diets and exercises, and by providing massage and a few selected drugs.

History tells us of remarkable cures performed by the early Christians. Faith and prayer were added to potent suggestive factors such as anointment with oil and the laying-on-of-hands (Weatherhead, 1952, p. 81). Appolonius of Tyana, a pagan of the first century A.D., was among those who was reputed to have performed miraculous cures. Apollonius was said by his followers to have been the son of God, to have appeared to them after his death, and then to have ascended bodily into heaven (Durant, 1944, p. 526).

INTO THE MIDDLE AGES AND BEYOND

Prestigious emperors and kings also played an important role in suggestive healing during the late Roman empire and throughout the Middle Ages. The Roman emperor Vespasian (first century A.D.) was said to have healed the blind by applying his spit to their eyes. (Today the claim would probably be modified to the healing of hysterical blindness). Clovis the Frank (fifth century) is also reported to have performed "miracle cures." In fact, "the king's touch" became a tradition. Many English monarchs since the time of Edward the Confessor (eleventh century) as well as powerful rulers on the European continent were reputed to possess this ability. Among those who were said to heal through "the king's touch" were Louis IX in France (thirteenth century), Henry IV in England (early fifteenth century), and, most especially, Charles II (seventeenth century) who touched nearly 100,000 people (Weatherhead, 1952, p. 49). It is recorded that in 1684 such a large crowd thronged for the touch of Charles II that six were trampled to death (Ludwig, 1964). Perhaps this incident belongs to the tradition of iatrogenic disorders.

Miracle cures have been credited not only to powerful kings and charismatic religious leaders but also to physicians. Paracelsus (sixteenth century), for instance, was praised for his miraculous cures of leprosy, cholera, and cancer. His treatment methods were varied. They included diet and herbs, vibrations, bleeding, purging, prayer, spells, invocations, amulets, charms, and talismans. With the possible exception of diets and herbs, all of these methods would now be viewed as assisting self-healing processes through their "suggestive potency." As we have already seen, the process involves changing the ill person's orientation from the negative (fear, worry, hopelessness, resentment, guilt, tension, and so forth) to the positive (peace of mind, relaxation, expectancy of cure). Some aspects of Paracelsus' theory of illness and health (the hermetic theory) can be viewed as in line with contemporary holistic medicine and are thus surprisingly modern. Paracelsus saw health as harmony and disease as maladjustment. This maladjusted (diseased) state of the person was thought to be related to an unhealthy or abnormal mental attitude. He conceived of the physician as the servant of nature. The character and personality of the physician are more important than the specific treatments. The physician must personally be in harmony with nature in order to be an agent in the total healing process. Paracelsus also emphasized—as alert physicians do today—that the restorative power of nature can be hindered by drugs, and he urged his fellow physicians to go easy with them (Atkinson, 1956).

Those who attempted to heal in the name of Christ apparently were just as successful as those with the power of the throne behind them. Good documentation is available for the effectiveness of Valentine Greatrakes (seventeenth century), a retired veteran of Cromwell's army. Greatrakes attempted to heal by stroking the skin of the sufferer either gently or vigorously while crying, "God Almighty heal and strengthen you for Jesus' sake!" Eye-witness accounts claim that many individuals with practically every kind of ailment were healed by Greatrakes.

A century later, Father Gassner was also performing apparently miraculous cures by calling upon the name of Jesus. Speaking in Latin, he would summon the demons by name. Once assembled, the demons were exorcised, and the illness was thereby cured. His words would also at times induce convulsions in those he treated. Fortunately, however, his suggestions could also stop the convulsions. This treatment method came in for critical scrutiny. The King of Bavaria appointed an investigative commission. This commission did not deny that the effects were, in fact, produced, although it concluded that these same effects could be produced by another method. This alternative method was simpler, did not involve trafficking with demons, and was altogether more scientific in character. The method, in fact, was one that was being developed by a member of the investigative commission. With this man and his alternative method we open a new chapter in the history of healing.

HEALING ENERGIES

Anton Mesmer's predecessors such as Father Gassner conceptualized their suggestive healing in religious terms. Mesmer used suggestive procedures that were similar, but Mesmer was a physician and a highly educated man. Furthermore, he was living during the Enlightment, a period of exceptional intellectual activity. Newton's theory of gravity had permeated the intellectual world, Benjamin Franklin and others had started to test the properties of electricity, and Lavoisier was making great discoveries in chemistry. It was natural for Mesmer to interpret the healing phenomena in terms of the scientific concepts of his day. He believed that his procedures involved the transmission to the sick individual of an energy or fluid. This fluid was present throughout the universe; therefore, the healer had a tremendous resource to draw upon. The healer was a person who had an excess of the fluid or, as it has been remembered by history of "animal magnetism." This surplus would be transmitted to the person whose sickness proclaimed a deficiency of animal magnetism.

There were a variety of specific ways by which the healing fluid/energy/magnetism could be transmitted, according to Mesmer. When Mesmer was the rage of Paris in 1784, the transmission procedure was as follows: a group of about thirty people self-selected as patients would sit in silence around a circular oak cask about a foot high. Within the cask or tub were scatterings of powdered glass and iron filings. The peculiar construction of the cask had a distinct purpose, supposedly to collect the fluid or healing energy in somewhat the same way that the Leyden jar—which had already been invented—would collect electricity. The group atmosphere was also important. The patients raised each other's expectancy that healing events most certainly would occur. To receive the fluid, the patients would at times hold on to metal rods that protruded from the cask (*baquet*). To transmit the fluid, they would hold hands or touch each other (Ellenberger, 1965). The room itself was dark, surrounded by thick curtains. Music from a pianoforte or a harmonicum would come from another room.

Finally, Mesmer himself would enter the room. He had a variety of suggestive methods at his disposal. He might, for instance, slowly move an iron wand toward the patient until it touched at a painful or diseased area. The wand was, of course, expected to transmit the healing fluid. At times he looked the patient directly in the eyes while he made "passes" with his hands an inch or two over the patient's body. These passes were intended to spread the healing energy. There were both brief and extended periods during which Mesmer placed his hands on the patient, again to transmit the fluid. On other occasions, Mesmer or one of his assistants would sit close to the patient, knee against knee, while moving the hand slightly above the patient's body, just an inch or two away without touching.

A detailed description of these passes has been provided by Deleuze (1825). Mesmer had seated himself with the patient's knees between his own. He asked the patient not to analyze or criticize what was happening. Instead, the patient was to let go of all bothersome thoughts, anxieties, and fears. The original mesmerist allowed a few moments to bring himself to a "state of self-collectedness." Then he took hold of each of the patient's thumbs for about five minutes, or until they felt quite warm. Next, he carried out his first pass by bringing his hands a fraction of an inch above the patient's face and then moving them to the shoulders where they were held for about a minute. Mesmer then drew his hand down along the patient's arms and hands, touching lightly. This pass was repeated five or six times. Mesmer then placed his hands close by the patient's head and slowly brought them down over his face and neck to the chest and stomach area where they remained for about two minutes. He continued with a variety of different kinds of passes. These included passing his hand slowly over the patient's body from head to feet, behind the patient's shoulders, and slowly along the spine to his hips, thighs, and feet. When "magnetizing" by the long pass—moving his hands slowly from the patient's head to his feet—Mesmer believed he was dispersing the healing energy or fluid over the patient's body and that it would accumulate in those parts that needed it most.

What were the effects? Some of the patients were not influenced at all. Others were affected in various ways. A few would have coughing spells; others would experience sensations of hot or cold or vibrations, or any combination of these. Some of his patients would become highly aroused, and have spectacular "crises" (fits or convulsions).

It should be noted that Mesmer's passes were highly intimate and suggestive. Although few words were spoken, there was an intimate aspect to each of the passes since Mesmer was physically close, moved his hands close to and sometimes on the patient, felt the heat radiated by the patient while, at the same time, the patient felt the heat from Mesmer's hands, and so on. Furthermore, the passes were not made in an impersonal or mechanical way. On the contrary, Mesmer and many of his followers were compassionate, caring, and loving toward their patients. As Deleuze (1825) pointed out, the mesmerists not only believed strongly in their ability to help their patients but had "benevolent feelings" and "a disinterested desire to do good."

Mesmer's passes conveyed an implicit but strong message: "I will heal you. . . . You are now being healed by the energy I transmit to you. . . . You can now relax and have peace of mind. . . . You can let go of your fears and unhappiness. . . . I care about you." Shor (1979) has pointed out that the common meaning of the word *suggestion* is not strong enough to give the full flavor of Mesmer's influence. Shor noted that "far richer and more accurate characterizations are terms such as enthusiastic credence, exalted confidence, intense emotive excitement, firm expectancy of influence, faith healing, and charismatic personality which . . . refer to emotionally highly charged beliefs giving expression to core energies of personality" (1979, p. 30).

Mesmer and his followers claimed that they cured various types of pains, including headaches, neuralgias, sciatica, gout and other rheumatic afflictions, skin diseases, tumors, and asthma. Elliotson and later mesmerists who published their cases in the movement's new journal, *The Zoist*, claimed that they healed all the illnesses listed above, plus eye inflammation, amenorrhea, impotency, insanity, and more.

Two considerations should be kept in mind in evaluating these claims: (1) as already mentioned, most ailments do heal themselves within a period of time whether they are treated by one method or another, or left entirely untreated; and (2) since about 50 percent of the illnesses diagnosed at the present time are found to be *mis*diagnosed when they are closely inspected by the most expert physicians (Gross, 1966; Sander, 1963), we can reasonably conjecture that many diagnoses were also incorrect in Mesmer's day. Because of the misdiagnosis factor, then, some people might seem to recover from conditions they never had in the first place. Despite these provisos, a close reading of the mesmerists' case reports yields the impression that their efforts did have effects. Individuals with a wide variety of both chronic and acute ailments were helped to recover more quickly through their interaction with a mesmeric healer. Some of these people had conditions that could be labeled as hysterical or psychosomatic (not that these labels explain very much), but not all could be fairly classified as such.

Several investigative commissions looked closely at the mesmeric methods (just as Mesmer had helped to investigate the earlier work of Father Gassner). In 1784 the king of France appointed selected members of the Academy of Sciences to evaluate Mesmer's method. The commission included Benjamin Franklin, then the United States ambassador, the great chemist Lavoisier, the ill-fated Dr. Guillotin who was later to fall victim to his own invention during the French Revolution, and the famous astronomer Bailly, among other notables. The commission worked with Deslon, a follower of Mesmer, who provided them with five people who had been found highly susceptible to animal magnetism. The first controlled or "single-blind" psychological experiment was performed on them by the commissioners. At times, the blind-folded participants were exposed to the healing fluid and at times they were not exposed. During some of the exposures they were told that they were receiving the fluid, and during other exposures they were not told they were receiving it. To complete the experimental design, they were sometimes told that they were receiving the treatment when, in fact, they were not. Clear-cut results were obtained. The participants felt the fluid or energy and were affected by it when they *believed* the treatment was being given. Whether or not the fluid was being transmitted made no difference; their beliefs were all that counted. There was no self-perceived effect of animal magnetism when the treatment was given without being identified as such.

The royal commission also observed how mesmeric procedures were used in the treatment of a larger number of patients. They concluded that the results were not brought about by a new form of energy or fluid but by psychological factors. They applied the words *imagination* and *imitation* to the psychological processes at work. Physical touch was also considered to play a role in arousing and exciting the patients. The commission also prepared a secret report to the king which noted that the close contact between the male mesmeric healer and the female patients often had strong sexual overtones.

Mesmerism was such a dramatic phenomenon and such a troubling one to the professional and scientific establishment that a second commission was appointed by the Royal Society of Medicine. The findings were much the same: the effects were caused by psychological factors, not some unknown energy or fluid. The official report emphasized that the effectiveness of the mesmeric healing procedures had been exaggerated. The procedures were said not to be effective when the disease could be clearly diagnosed and had a known etiology. The effect of mesmerism, according to the commission, occurred when the disease was minor and the symptoms ambiguous. The Royal Society of Medicine's commission identified the probable effective agents in what success mesmerism did yield: (1) the arousal of hope and expectations of recovery, and (2) the abstinence from medicines or remedies previously taken. The first factor is congruent with the modern viewpoint that sick individuals recover more quickly when they feel that something is being done for them. The second factor is consistent with another modern view, namely, that all drugs have a variety of effects on the body, some of which are harmful and some of which can be helpful. All drugs can give rise to side effects, some severe. Therefore, a substantial proportion of patients improve when they are instructed to stop taking all their medications (Gross, 1966).

The verdict of two distinguished commissions did not deter all the followers of Mesmer. Men such as Puysegur, Deleuze, Elliotson, and Esdaile continued to adhere to the theory of animal magnetism, and these "fluidists" pursued their practice throughout France and other parts of Europe, and later in the United States and other nations. Puysegur, a nobleman, made a discovery that in retrospect can be seen as the beginning of another significant element of the healing tradition. He was using mesmeric passes with a man by the name of Victor Race, one of the nobleman's own peasants. Race closed his eyes during the procedure and appeared to be asleep. Nevertheless, he spoke very intelligently while in this state (of what now might be termed altered consciousness) and responded to various instructions and suggestions. This was perhaps the first intermix of suggestions for healing with an apparent sleep-like condition (hypnosis, as it was to be called).

Some of the post–Mesmer animal magnetists, however, did take a lesson from the commissions' findings, which also coincided with some of their own experiences. This new generation of healers made more use of verbal suggestions, and less of passes and other nonverbal procedures. One of the first to make this switch was the Abbe Faria (1755–1819), who had concluded that the mesmeric procedures could be viewed as nonverbal suggestions (Dingwall, 1967, p. 34). Mesmer's touchings, laying-on-of-hands, and passes were suggesting ideas to the patient such as, "I care about you and I can heal you. Be at peace about your ailment. Relax and have hope, because you will be well." Although Faria still continued to use some passes, his primary techniques were verbal. He first commanded the patient to sleep and then gave suggestions that aimed—quite directly—to relieve the ailments: "You will sleep calmly and peacefully at night. . . . You will wake up in the morning feeling very refreshed. . . . The pain will become less and less, and then will go away entirely."

By 1841, a Scottish surgeon was writing about the psychological factors in mesmerism. James Braid dropped the term mesmerism and replaced it with a new term of his own devising: *neurohypnotism.* This was later shortened to the *hypnotism* that has become a familiar, yet frequently misunderstood term. Braid's viewpoint continued to evolve as he applied hypnosis to his patients. He finally arrived at the conclusion that patients are influenced both by nonverbal and verbal suggestions "according to their expectation or belief." He no longer believed that his own concept, hypnosis, was an accurate representation of the suggestion process, but the term was already proving popular and could not be successfully recalled and shelved by its creator.

Early in his research, Braid would start his procedure by asking the patient to look up at a small bright object held about ten or twelve inches above the middle of his forehead. This procedure caused the patient to turn his eyes upward, which was a strain that often produced a "trancey" or dizzy feeling. At first, Braid interpreted the eye-fixation procedure as having its effect through fatiguing the levator muscle of the eye. Later, however, he observed that the effects were ambiguous and inconsistent when the patient did not know what to expect. Consequently, Braid concluded that psychological factors were the important ones. After the preliminary state-inducing procedures, Braid would give his patients direct verbal suggestions for healing, health, and well-being. Detailed case histories were presented in his text. These indicated that suggestions (usually given over a series of sessions) were markedly helpful in the treatment of rheumatism, torticollis (wry neck), migraine, epilepsy, deafness, nearsightedness, strabismus, and other ailments. Some of the diagnoses were probably invalid, and others might have involved hystero-epilepsy and hysterical deafness instead of organic disturbance. Nevertheless, a review of these cases indicates that verbal suggestions as used by Braid were remarkably effective in helping a wide variety of ill and impaired individuals.

Within a generation, Liebeault and then Bernheim had published a large number of detailed cases that demonstrated the effects of direct verbal suggestions on a broad spectrum of diseases. Bernheim had a somewhat different way of interpreting the phenomena. He emphasized that his suggestions improved the patient's condition when they opposed or altered the patient's *self*-suggestion. It was the patient's own pattern of thoughts that were producing, maintaining, or exacerbating the illness. According to Bernheim, hypnotic induction was just one more suggestion which, when accepted by the patient, helped him become more responsive to other suggestions. It was not that something quite powerful and exotic existed in the trance. Rather, the important thing was that the patient believed he was asleep or in a special state that would make healing possible. Although he made use of sleep suggestions himself at times, Bernheim did not find this procedure to be essential. Patients were also responsive to therapeutic suggestions when they were not given sleep or hypnotic instructions. Many individuals were highly responsive to suggestions without going through the hypnotic procedure, while there were some for whom hypnosis did not enhance responsiveness to subsequent suggestions.

Bernheim would induce the sleep or hypnotic state with instructions such as these: "Look at me and think of nothing but sleep. Your eyelids begin to feel heavy. Your eyes are tired. They begin to wink. They are getting moist. You cannot see distinctly. . . . Your lids are closing. You cannot open them again. Your arms feel heavy; so do your legs. You cannot feel anything. Your hands are motionless. You see nothing. You are going to sleep. Sleep!" Next, Bernheim would give direct suggestions for therapeutic improvement. Sometimes they would be specific: "You can now move the (paralyzed) arm." Sometimes they would be more general: "You will get well. Your state will improve. You will become calm at first, less frightened, then stronger. Your aches will grow less; the pains will grow less. Gradually the muscles will loosen up. Your joints will be less stiff. Your limbs will become stronger and stronger."

The following conclusions emerge as one reads carefully through Bernheim's (1887, 1891) texts and, especially, through his detailed case presentations:

1. Bernheim had enormous *prestige* in the eyes of his patients. He was the head of the service, and a professor. His marked prestige, however, derived not only from his broad knowledge and expertise, but also from his manner and his level of being. Bernheim was a kind, mature person who functioned at a high level and therefore was himself perhaps his most valuable instrument of treatment.

2. Bernheim was a *compassionate* and *caring* person who was devoted to helping his patients.

3. Bernheim *varied his approach* and his suggestions to fit the patient. He talked to his patients personally and intimately. He gave therapeutic suggestions either with or without prior sleep induction depending upon the person and the situation. To some patients he deliberately gave nonverbal suggestions by administering electricity, massage, cold, heat, and other physical stimuli which implicitly carried the suggestion, "This physical procedure is powerful and it will heal you."

4. In the same basic way as his predecessors who used suggestions (Faria, Braid, Liebault), Bernheim *ameliorated* a large variety of illnesses. The partial or complete cures that appeared to follow his forceful suggestions included not only hystero-epilepsy and other apparently hysterical illnesses but also enuresis, insomnia, sonambulism, and illnesses that superficially seem more "organic" (e.g., rheumatism, dysmenorrhea, chronic gastritis, epigastric pain, thoracic pain, sciatica, and tic douloureux).

Other physicians of Bernheim's time also used suggestive procedures knowledgeably in their treatment (for instance, Delbouef, 1886; Forel, 1907; Wetterstrand, 1891), as did the next generation (for example, Bramwell, 1903; Janet, 1919). These clinicians also reported that verbal therapeutic suggestions, given with or without suggestions to sleep, were much more useful in medicine then they at first expected.

Despite a marked decline in the publicity received by suggestive or hypnotic therapy during the first half of the twentieth century, there does not seem to have been any decline in the actual number of physicians who were using these methods. The proportion of physicians making regular and knowledgeable use of suggestive techniques seemed to have been relatively small during the nineteenth century, and there were always a few more ready to carry forward this tradition. During this period, hypnotherapy or suggestive therapy was used in England by Hadfield, Brown, and others; in the Soviet Union by Behkterev; and in the United States by Schilder, Kubie, Gill, Erickson, and many others. During the 1950s, however, there was a decided increase in the United States in the number of physicians who attended workshops which aimed to teach the use of suggestions in therapy. During this period, Erickson, Kroger, Schneck, Kline, Watkins, and others crossed the nation to present workshops on suggestive therapy or hypnosis. During the 1960s and 70s, a series of useful texts appeared on clinical uses of hypnosis (Cheek and Lebron, 1968; Crasilneck & Hall, 1975; Erickson, 1967; Hartland, 1966; Kroger, 1963; Kroger & Fezler, 1976; Meares, 1960; Schneck, 1965). Hypnosis had become an acceptable part of the medical armamentarium.

NONVERBAL HEALING AFTER MESMER

We have seen that some therapists, typically those working in medical settings, saw the effectiveness of mesmeric procedures as the consequence of psychological factors and began using more and more verbal suggestions. This tradition became known as suggestive therapy and hypnotism. However, another group of individuals continued to use the procedures that became famous with Mesmer (but most of which had long preceded him). These healers typically did not work in medical settings. They dealt in passes, touching, and prolonged contact, or laying-on-of-hands. Sometimes these procedures were conceptualized in mesmeric terms: that is, the healer was thought to be a conduit for transmitting healing energy to the sick individual. Not all of these healers retained (or even understood) the whole quasi-scientific vision Mesmer had elaborated around his procedures, but the core concept of energy transmission remained.

There were other conceptualizations as well. Some healers operated within a religious context, their energy associated with the Divine. Still other healers agreed in part with the mesmeric formulation but added one or both of the following beliefs: (1) departed spirits guided their healing (*spiritualist* or *spiritist* healing); (2) their own psychic abilities were guiding the healing (*psychic* healing). Although healers differed in their viewpoints, when they were at work there were at least two major characteristics in common: they had the intention of helping the patient, and they felt that they gave of themselves or of their own energy in helping the patient regain health.

The charismatic healing tradition did not die with Greatrakes, Gasner, and other eighteenth century workers of the miracle cure. In the United States during the 1880s, for example, Father Schlatter was reputed to have healed through touch. To extend his reach, he mailed handkerchiefs that he had touched to sick people throughout the nation. Unfortunately, we will never know whether or not these "miraclized" handkerchiefs might have proved effective because the U.S. Post Office quickly stepped in and stopped the practice.

One of the most socially significant consequences of the charismatic healing tradition in the United States was its role in the creation of a new religious movement. Phineas P. Quimby, a watchmaker by trade, witnessed a French mesmerist performing his passes at a show in Maine. Charles Poyen (1837) influenced several dozen New Englanders to take up this practice, with Quimby the star pupil. Quimby, however, had an original and inquisitive mind and soon left mesmerism behind. He came to the conclusion that what we call disease is produced by the individual's state of mind or beliefs. He emphasized strongly the power of belief: when a person recovered from illness the healing work had been done not by the medicine but by the physician–patient mutual belief system. Quimby gained a wide reputation as a healer. However, he steadfastly rejected the idea (current then as now) that psychic or other strange forces were operating. Although he would rub the patient's head or gently manipulate a disabled limb, Quimby regarded these actions as a concession to the need for the patient to see something happening. The real treatment consisted in the dialogue and the relationship.

One of his patients was a forty-five-year-old bedridden and apparently helpless woman. Quimby's ministrations had a dramatic effect on Mary Baker Eddy. After her paralysis was overcome, she rewrote his manuscripts and published them under her own name. *Science and Health with Key to the Scriptures* (1875) became the bible of what was not only a new method of healing but a new religion — Christian Science. A basic dogma of Christian Science (Eddy, not Quimby version) is that all disease is unreal because it is a delusion of the "mortal mind." This belief has resulted in an unknown number of deaths because physicians were not consulted (Janet, 1919; Weatherhead, 1952). The denial of illness, however, is not always a negative factor. While denial increases the risk in life-threatening illness, it can facilitate recovery from the great majority of diseases that are affected by the recuperative powers of the body. As Weatherhead has observed:

> Suffice it to say here that the power of the mind over the body is such that, again and again, the treatment of the Christian Science healer, in spite of the faulty philosophy which we have examined, has brought health. When fear and all other unhealthy and negative emotions are banished; when disease is minimized and the thought of the patient is turned away from himself and his sad plight, to the splendour and joy of God; when recovery is believed not merely to be possible, but imminent, psychological conditions are set up within the ego which give the healing force of Nature the maximum opportunity (1952, pp. 181–182).

The potency of suggestive and psychological factors has been acknowledged by some religiously oriented healers. Elwood Worcester and Rev. McComb, founders of the influential Emmanuel movement, believed that healing results from persuasion and suggestion. These processes are thought to operate through the subconscious. The stability and calm that accompanies surrender to God also facilitates healing. The sense of oneness with God was seen as exercising a soothing influence on the central nervous system, resulting in a general sense of serenity that provides an ideal climate for healing.

The importance of suggestion is mentioned occasionally in the written work of contemporary healers. The healer's love and concern for the patient receives much more emphasis, however. Some have also underscored the importance of the healer "uniting" with the patient. Rev. Edgar Jackson, for example, sees himself as a catalyst or stimulator. By holding the patient "in loving concern," he stimulates the recuperative functions (Kruger, 1974, pp. 311–312). The care and compassion transmitted to the patient are accompanied by an enhanced expectancy of cure. There are implicit and explicit suggestions of recovery. Rev. Jackson, one of the most respected contemporary healers, states that the methods used by himself and others do involve strong suggestive or placebo effects but that these have always played an important role in both medical and nonmedical healing.

The contention that healing is based primarily on love from the healer is ably presented by Father Roy Hendricks of the Order of St. Luke. He states that the essence of his healing procedures (which include meditation, prayer, laying-on-of-hands, and anointing with oil) is "loving people" (Kruger, 1974, pp. 275–276). He sees the laying-on-of-hands as symbolic. The real cure is self-inspired. The patient's outlook changes, and this makes recuperation of the body possible. It is a three-phase procedure, then: (1) love and symbolic action by the healer, leading to (2) a more affirmative psychological orientation in the patient, which in turn induces (3) a physiological state favorable for recovery.

Investigators who have studied lay healers have reached similar conclusions. E.N. Shealy (1975) brought healers into his medical clinic to observe their effectiveness. He found that those who helped the patients were characterized by two closely related traits: they were loving individuals who were also very sincere in their desire to help others. Psychologists Krippner and Villoldo (1976) studied the methods and effectiveness of various types of healers, concluding that the characteristics of a good healer are the same as those Carl Rogers had found in good psychotherapists: empathy, warmth, genuineness. Krippner and Villoldo see these characteristics, especially the genuine concern or love of healers for their patients, as effective because hope and recuperative resources are mobilized. LeShan's studies led him to a similar conclusion: the sick person is aided in his recovery when he feels totally loved (LeShan, 1979). The effective healer allows his love and caring to flow and become one with the patient. This interpersonal unity is said to far transcend our ordinary level of intimacy.

Delores Krieger (1979) is still another who has arrived at a similar conclusion. In her case, this was based on her efforts to teach one of the traditional healing techniques (laying-on-of-hands) to a rather large number of nurses. She concluded that the effective healer has a strong motivation to help others and a strong emotional involvement with the patient. This is virtually undistinguishable from the finding in Meck's (1977) study that successful healers are "almost invariably warm, loving people with a great concern for their patients."

The successful healer's loving concern is a theme also highlighted by other writers. Weatherhead concluded in his classic work, *Psychology, Religion, and Healing* (1952), that the most important factors in religious healing are love from the healer and faith on the part of the patient that he will recover. Well known healers in England, who are practicing at the present time, formulate the important factors along similar lines. Harry Edwards emphasizes compassion and sympathy, together with the willingness to give of oneself to others. Gordon Turner also sees the critical variables as compassion and love which lead to an "attunement" or merging of the personalities of the healer and the patient.

In summary, there is broad agreement that effective healers are compassionate people who care deeply about their patients and have a strong desire to help them. At least part of their effectiveness seems to derive from the healing power of love. This term is quite old-fashioned. Perhaps medical, psychological, and social sciences have now approached a state of knowledge at which this term can be fully appreciated, as will be suggested later in this chapter. Emerson (1965) wrote of love as the one remedy for all ills, the panacea of nature. Sorokin (1954) held that the spontaneous self-giving of total concern that we call love is literally a life-giving force and, at the same time, the best therapy. Fromm (1956) argued that the deepest need of man is for love to remove him from the prison of his aloneness in the world. These observers, and many others through the years, have been telling us the truth. At times their messages have been taken as though rhetorical exercises or sentimental indulgences. It has been assumed that the real factors at work must be mechanistic. These will be revealed to us eventually through detailed analyses and will be dubbed with properly objective scientific names. It seems to us that there are, indeed, processes at work that can be regarded as mechanisms. And yet the key words may turn out to be some of the most familiar in our language, *love* being the foremost. Love can enhance recuperative powers by reducing isolation, hopelessness and fear, and by increasing serenity or peace of mind. These processes are not afloat in a nebulous, linguistic universe, but are close to the very breath of our life. We will return to these considerations after examining another aspect of healing: the development of the medical sciences.

DEVELOPMENT OF THE MEDICAL SCIENCES

Up to this point, we have focused primarily on suggestive therapy and lay healing. These approaches have been helpful in alleviating illness, sometimes dramatically. During the past few centuries, however, the medical sciences have gained such substantial new knowledge that today the physician can make a valid claim for superiority over the suggestive therapist or the lay healer. We will be offering the view that the most effective healers of the future will combine the suggestive potency of the best hypnotist, the love and compassion of the best lay healers, and the knowledge of the human body in health and disease that is associated with the best physician. Before presenting this argument, however, it is necessary to review at least a few of the major developments that have occurred in the medical sciences during recent centuries.

Medicine's remarkable advances in the present and past century were preceded by the painstaking work of Vesalius (circa 1543) in dissecting and describing human anatomy, the breakthrough of William Harvey (circa 1628) in tracing the circulation of the blood through the body, and the ingenuity of Edward Jenner (circa 1798) in developing the first vaccination (against smallpox). Significant developments continued during the next several generations. William Beaumont (circa 1833) observed the functioning stomach of a wounded trapper and came up with the first modern description of the digestive process. Johannes Muller clarified many of the body's functions in his profound *Handbook of Human Physiology* (1834–1840). Claude Bernard (circa 1865) founded modern experimental physiology while clarifying the processes of digestion, glycogen metabolism, and vasomotor changes. Rudolf Virchow (circa 1858) demonstrated the role of the cell in pathological changes, while Herman von Helmholtz (circa 1859) and others were clarifying the physiological processes associated with vision and audition.

Perhaps the most important developments were the formulation, confirmation, and successful application of the *germ theory* of disease, which might be considered the greatest advance in healing that has occurred at any point in human history. Applications of the germ theory have either eradicated or markedly reduced the prevalence of many diseases that have afflicted people throughout the centuries— smallpox, syphilis, gonorrhea, tuberculosis, typhoid, plague, malaria, yellow fever, and more. The theory that some diseases are caused by nonobservable micro-organisms (germs) received strong experimental support when Louis Pasteur (1822–1895) demonstrated that fermentation was produced by living organisms. Pasteur then applied this concept to show how anthrax and rabies could be prevented. Also important in understanding disease in terms of microorganisms was Joseph Lister's (circa 1865) demonstration that surgery could be made safer by antiseptic measures which prevented wound infection, and Ignaz Philipp Semmelweis' similar conclusion with regard to obstetrics.

The procession of germ theory triumphs was well underway by 1882 when Robert Koch discovered the tubercle bacillus. Two decades later Paul Ehrlich demonstrated that arsphenamine could destroy the syphilis micro-organism in the human body. By 1928, Alexander Fleming had discovered the antibiotic (germ-killing) properties of penicillin. The potent sulfonamide drugs appears in the late 1930s, and a decade later a host of new anitbiotics, such as streptomycin, were proving their effectiveness. Advances in immunology led to methods for combating invading microorganisms in other ways: typhoid vaccine, tetanus, and diphtheria antitoxins, and viral vaccines for yellow fever, poliomyelitis, and influenza. Micro-organisms responsible for malaria, yellow fever, and other diseases were controlled by identifying and eliminating the insects responsible for transmitting them to humans. The germ theory, then, led to victories over a variety of life-threatening illnesses through stimulating the development of antibiotics, the developing of vaccines and antitoxins, and utilizing preventive measures in the environment.

Although the control of diseases associated with micro-organisms has been the most powerful accomplishment of modern medicine, other important advances have also been made:

1. The expansion of *endoctrinological knowledge* has had direct treatment applications. These successes began with Murray's (1891) use of thyroid extract for the treatment of myxedema. Other signifi-

cant applications included Banting and Best's (1921) discovery of insulin and its usefulness in diabetes, the utilization of cortisone to control rheumatoid arthritis and as a general anti-inflammatory agent, and the development of contraceptive pills based on improved knowledge of the sex hormones. These are but a few of the practical applications from the expansion of endocrinological knowledge, and, of course, research and clinical trials in this area continue vigorously today.

2. Knowledge of *vitamins* and their role in metabolism has greatly improved. This led to the control of rickets, scurvy, beriberi, and other debilitating ailments.

3. Dramatic advances have been made in *surgery* and the underlying science of *anesthesiology*. Anesthesiology has progressed steadily from the first use of ether in 1842 by Crawford Long to the introduction of cyclopropane (1933), the development of intravenous anesthesia, the introduction of curare to produce muscular paralysis, and numerous other additions to the anesthesia spectrum. Surgery's progress has been no less remarkable. This progress was stimulated by the development of methods for combating infections by antisepsis (destruction of micro-organisms) and later by asepsis (avoidance of contamination). Highlights in surgical history include the development of blood transfusions to combat shock, the introduction of the operating microscope, and the development of abdominal and open-heart surgery, bypass operations, neurosurgery, plastic surgery, organ transplantation, and procedures for repair or replacement of damaged or worn-out tissues with plastics and other foreign material.

We have now reviewed some of the highlights in the three traditions of medicine, suggestive therapy, and lay healing. Each approach has strengths and weaknesses. The ideal modern healer would integrate the strengths of all. This ideal healer would be thoroughly acquainted with all the basic medical sciences: anatomy, physiology, bacteriology, pathology, pharmacology, and so forth. These sciences provide the useful perspective of the human organism as a complex body comprised of cells, tissues, and organs. The human organism answers to this description, but such a description is quite incomplete. The human being is a mind–body unity; therefore, the complementary perspective, which sees health and disease as related to the thoughts and emotions of the person, is equally necessary. This integrative or holistic perspective requires more emphasis than it has usually received during the rise of scientific medicine with its revelations on the biological level.

There is another topic that also requires more emphasis: the *self-healing capacities* of the organism. Many relevant data are now available, and more can be expected, but seldom have the facts of psychobiological functioning been examined systematically from the standpoint of their self-healing implications.

In the next two sections, we examine these topics: self-healing capacities, and the effects that our thoughts and emotions have on health and illness. These considerations are essential in understanding the effects of the three approaches, and the necessity of their being incorporated in the training of ideal healers.

CREATION AND SURVIVAL OF THE ORGANISM

The living organism is an amazing fact of nature, a fact that becomes all the more amazing the more closely we examine it. Without some appreciation of the normal miracles involved in creation and maintenance of the organism, we cannot hope to understand healing interventions of any type. Attention will be given, then, to a few of the awesome processes through which the organism is constructed, maintained, repaired, and healed.

Creation of the Organism

Most educated people today have read about the processes that form the human being. Fewer of us, however, appreciate the magnificence of these processes. The fertilized egg is already the product of goal-directed processes in both the sperm and egg which have insured that each party has but half the chromosomes of its parent organism. The amount of *information* present in the fertilized egg is so vast that one is almost lost in trying to grasp its precision and density. This information, which serves as blueprints, plans, and programs for forming a new human being, is far more extensive than the information contained on all the pages of the *Encyclopedia Britannica*. The human being is comprised of trillions of cells, each of which carries out organized chemical processes which must harmonize with those processes in its trillions of neighbors. These multitudinous and complex processes all must be specified in the information transmitted by the genetic code. The information transmitted from the parents must specify how these chemical processes are to be formed in the countless cells of the body, and then how they are to be maintained over the life span of the organism. This information, all contained in a particular configuration in mini-microscopic scale, must also specify how the cells are to organize themselves into tissues, the tissues into organs, and the organs in to the integrated organism.

We cannot even begin to describe all the harmonious processes that go on microscopically to form a human being (and it cannot be said that all the processes are known today). It may be sufficient to say here that the relatively large fertilized egg divides many, many times to form a large number of small cells. These microscopic entities then migrate, change, and coalesce in a harmonious way to form the varied tissues of our body. Billions upon billions of cells formed in one part of the egg move harmoniously to another part of the growing organism. As they migrate, they also change in form and function. If we look, for example, at the migrating cells which are to become part of the nervous system, we see one changing into a neuroglia, another into a cell with many dendrites, and still another into a cell with few dendrites and a very long axon. As the nerve cells form and migrate, they also unite, coalesce, and interdigitate with each other and with other kinds of cells (for instance, those that will form blood vessels). This union of different types of cells will form the brain, spinal cord, peripheral nerves, and other parts of the nervous system. Other groups of cells are formed in a similar way and the results are the multitude of smooth muscle cells in our ever-pumping heart, the many miles of cells that comprise our capillaries and other blood vessels, and all other structures that comprise our body.

It is possible to describe these processes up to a point. We can describe how some of the cells are formed and how they change into markedly different types of cells with entirely different functions. One becomes an elongated kidney cell that specializes in removing only the undesirable products from the blood. Another becomes a striated muscle cell that produces bodily movements when it contracts in response to a specific chemical stimulus from a nerve. Still another cell that seemed to start its life in a common, undifferentiated form ends up as a retinal rod cell that emits electrical impulses when stimulated by light. We can also describe — up to a point — how cells migrate to just the right place and coalesce in just the right way to serve just the right functions for the integrated organism. Yet it is far beyond our limited comprehension to say in any fundamental sense how these awesomely complex and yet harmoniously purposive processes come about.

What do these processes have to do with healing? The wondrous processes that formed the organism do not suddenly stop. They continue in an altered form to maintain the organism, to keep it functioning harmoniously, and to repair or heal in the event of injury or malfunctioning. When the organism has been "constructed," when each kind of cell is functioning in its proper location, the cells continue to multiply and reform themselves in response to aging and damage. Some cells are continually being used, sloughed off, or destroyed and are continually, every moment of our lives, in the process of being remade. These include the epidermal cells of the skin, the red cells in the blood, the cells lining the intestinal tract and the very different cells lining the cornea of the eye, the sperm cells, and others. If pathogenic bacteria or viruses invade the organism, designated cells will either manufacture specific chemicals to destroy the invaders or themselves move into direct combat. Highly specialized and coordinated operations also occur when the organism is wounded or a bone is broken.

Processes of maintenance, repair, and healing go on at every moment of our lives. We will examine some of these known but neglected processes in order to develop the necessary context for the various types of healing interventions that have been reviewed.

Self-Healing of Cuts and Wounds

All arteries, arterioles, veins, and venules contain microscopic muscle cells that narrow the vessel when they contract. What happens when we suffer a cut? The first major reaction involves these tiny muscle cells. They contract and pull the blood vessels as tight as possible to slow down the blood loss. Next, a sticky substance is secreted from the damaged ends of the blood vessels. This substance helps the blood vessels cohere together. As these (and other) events are slowing the flow of blood through the wounds, chemicals are released that will produce coagulation. These blood-clotting chemicals are emitted from cells at the surface of the cut itself, and also from cell-like particles (platelets) that flow along with the blood and adhere to the surface of a cut.

The chemical component of the healing process is itself orchestrated in fine detail. The first chemical molecule that is released reacts with another that is always present in the blood (Factor A) and converts this into an enzyme (catalyst). The newly created enzyme then reacts with another chemical molecule (Factor B) that is also present in the blood. Factor B becomes transformed into another enzyme—and on and on it goes. This cascade-like chain reaction continues for at least thirteen steps. In other words, a newly created enzyme reacts with a chemical in the blood to convert it into another enzyme which then reacts with another blood chemical to convert it into still another enzyme, and so on. If we skip ahead to the eleventh step of the reaction, prothromblin is converted into thrombin. Fibrinogen, which has been present in the blood all this time, is transformed by thrombin into a particular type of fibrous molecule known as fibrin. The fibrin molecules then line up in adherence to each other until they extend continuously across the cut ends of the injured blood vessel. This forms a fibrous network which looks like a complex spider web. The red cells floating in the blood become attached to this fibrous network as though it were a sticky net. Platelets also attach to the fibrin/red blood cell net. This net—together with the red blood cells and platelets it has "captured"—constitutes the *clot* which prevents the wounded person from bleeding to death.

The body's repair and healing work does not stop here. The platelets, utilizing their pseudopodia (false feet), pull on the fibrin molecules to tighten them. The tightened net (comprised of fibrin, red blood cells, and platelets) is the *scab*, the final step in the process of blood coagulation.

After the scab is formed, there is still the necessity for the cut tissue to reform itself, to return to its whole, pre-traumatic condition. The epithelial cells on the edge of the wound begin to divide and multiply, and then to migrate into the wound area to form the new skin. This process is accomplished in a complex and ingenious way. The new skin has to form beneath the scab. The cells that are waiting to multiply and form the new skin themselves secrete powerful enzymes. These chemicals dissolve the scab on its underside. As the new skin takes its place it proves to be comprised of the same cellular layers as the skin it replaces. The cells are arranged in the same complex configuration. The epidermis, the dermis, the layer of fat underlying the skin, the blood vessels, the nerve fibers, the sweat glands, and the skin hairs all are reformed in a goal-directed way, so they are the same as the previous version.

Self-Healing of Bone Fractures

The organism repairs a broken bone in the same goal-directed way it repairs a wound. In fact, the blood vessels in the damaged bone begin to form a clot (hematoma) by utilizing the same thirteen-step cascading reaction described above. While this chain reaction is in progress, "eating cells" (phagocytes) migrate to the area of crushed bone tissue. They clean the debris by ingesting the tiny bone fragments. The next action is the responsibility of osteoblasts—bone cells that do nothing else but migrate to fracture areas and manufacture new bone. The osteoblasts first remove specific amino acides from the blood. The amino acids are then worked upon by the osteoblasts to create a large protein molecule: collagen. The busy osteoblasts also commandeer calcium from the blood and attach these molecules to the collagen. The collagen-calcium molecules are then secreted by the osteoblasts, another set of chemical reactions is performed, and behold: *bone!*

The osteoblasts not only rebuild the bone; they also remodel it. As the bone begins to heal, the alignment may be off. The osteoblasts will then remodel it until good alignment is achieved. A surgeon is not always able to place the ends of broken bones into a straight alignment. The organism itself compensates, then does its own remodelling so that the bones will be straight when healed (Nolan, 1974). This process of compensatory remodelling is especially efficient in children. In elderly individuals, however, this process is much less efficient, and serious problems can be created.

The efficiency of both wound and bone healing varies among individuals. Age plays a role, but "general health and happiness" are significant factors at all ages. The healing process moves faster and more efficiently when the individual is in a positive state of mind. By contrast, the condition that is called depression (an ambiguous and, in some respects, controversial term) can be pervasive. The depressed orientation (for want of a better term) is manifest in every part of the person—in the chemical molecules that coagulate the blood, in the cells that rebuild cutaneous tissue, in the osteoblasts that rebuild bone, as well as in the other trillions of body cells.

Self-Defense: The Immune System

The organism can be viewed as a vast nation comprised of trillions of citizens (cells) which are organized into systems of transportation (circulation), waste-disposal (kidney, bladder, urethra, and so on), communication (nervous and endocrine systems), chemical factories (liver), and defense (the immune system), to name some of the more obvious. The immune system plays an essential role in defending the organism both from its own lawless citizens (cancer cells) and from foreign invaders such as disease-producing bacteria. The functions of the immune system are very important for understanding the nature of self-healing processes. How the immune system works is of equal importance in understanding why healers of all types (medical, suggestive, and psychic or religious healers) do *not* themselves heal the sick individual. What happens is that drugs, suggestions, and psycho-spiritual effects stimulate and accelerate the individual's own self-defense and self-healing processes.

The immune system possesses at least three kinds of defense forces: (1) phagocytes that destroy invaders by ingesting or eating them; (2) antibodies that destroy pathogenic bacterial cells in somewhat the same way a torpedo destroys a battleship; and (3) the system of T cells which destroy pathogenic cells by injecting lethal chemicals into them. Each of these systems will be described briefly.

The first immunological defense system is comprised of phagocytes, white blood cells that protect us primarily from bacterial and viral invaders. Although most noticeable in the blood stream, they also patrol many other tissues throughout the body. There are about 200 billion phagocytes in our body. Multiply each person in the United States by 1,000, and we have some idea of their abundance within our own body. When a phagocyte has been alerted to the presence of a bacterium, virus, or other invading micro-organism within its vicinity, it moves toward the alien like a tiny amoeba. The invader is engulfed. Once inside the phagocyte, the invader is doused with enzymes and then digested. The invader probably brought about its own destruction by chemically telegraphing its approach to the ever-alert phagocytes.

The antibody-antigen reaction is the second immunological defense system. This goes into action when invading pathogenes are detected by a special type of white blood cell, the messenger lymphocytes. These are constantly on patrol. The messenger lymphocytes move toward the bacteria. They touch and inspect them, determining what specific chemicals (antigens) characterize the invader. This information is conveyed to other white blood cells (B lymphocytes). These latter cells are found in the lymph nodes. The B lymphocytes then start building specific molecules (antibodies) that fit the chemical configuration of the invading bacteria like a key into a lock. The anitbody molecules are made by each B lymphocyte at the incredible rate of 125,000 per second. They are crafted to attack and destroy only the specific bacteria that has been identified as the invader. At no point is this a simple process. To destroy each bacterium, the antibody molecules need the assistance of nine different types of protein molecules that are always present in the blood (all these together are known as complement). Complement lines up with the specific antibody molecules that have attached to the bacterial wall and, acting in concert, they literally blow a hole in the bacterium and destroy it.

Our third immunological defense system revolves around another type of white blood cell, the T cell. T cells are found in the lymph nodes (as are the B cells already discussed). They receive information from the messenger lymphocytes. As soon as information has been received from the messenger, the T cell transforms itself. It enlarges, becomes engorged with enzymes, and moves out of the lymph node to attack the enemy. The target of T cells is not bacteria, but intracellular pathogens such as viruses, cancer cells, and cells from a foreign tissue or organ (such as a transplant). The T cell touches the cancer (or other foreign) cell and shoots enzymes that destroy the enemy structure.

The Organism and the Healer

There are limits to the effectiveness of the immune system and all self-healing and repairing operations. Nevertheless, the major point must be emphasized as strongly as possible: the organism is constructed so as to maintain itself, fight off pathogens, and heal. The most important function for both medical and nonmedical healers is to help sick people heal themselves by stimulating the wound or bone repair system, the immunological system, and all other supportive systems such as the endocrine and nervous systems. Physicians can set bones, but the broken bones must heal themselves. Physicians can prescribe antibiotic drugs, but the drugs do not do the job themselves. They operate by slowing down the bacteria or viruses so that phagocytes, antibodies, and T cells can do their work more easily. In fact, all of the antibiotic drugs available in the world today would not enable a single person to survive if his immune system were not functioning (Glaser, 1976).

The organism is constructed with amazing know-how and resources for self-protection and healing. How well it carries out these functions, however, is affected by nutrition, exercise, and many other variables, including an all-encompassing variable that can be termed happiness. We maintain and heal ourselves better when we feel positive (happy, flowing, relaxed) then when we are negative (worried, depressed, unloved), as informed observers continue to note (Rogers, Dubey, & Reich, 1979).

This contention is supported by a wealth of research data. We will now examine some of the evidence for the view that negative thoughts and emotions can lead to and maintain disease.

DETRIMENTAL EFFECTS OF NEGATIVE THOUGHTS

A series of careful research studies indicate that a variety of illnesses may be causally related to such negative personal orientations as hopelessness, feeling unloved and unlovable, low self-esteem, and feeling guilty or angry (Lynch, 1977).

In one of the earlier and most celebrated studies of this type, Wolf and Wolff (1947) showed how negative feelings affect the stomach. They worked with Tom, a patient with a gastric fistula (an opening from the stomach to the body surface). They could look directly into Tom's stomach and did so in a wide variety of situations. Wolf and Wolff found that Tom's stomach functioning depended on his thoughts, feelings, and emotions. When Tom was angry, his stomach would become engorged with blood. As it became engorged (hyperemic), more acid would be secreted. His stomach would act in just the opposite way when Tom was sad or withdrawn. The blood would move away from the stomach (isochemia of gastric mucosa), and the acid secretions would stop. In brief, negative states such as anger and sadness lead to the kind of stomach malfunctioning that is associated with indigestion, gastritis, ulcers, and other disorders.

Kasl and Cobb (1970) found that a number of diseases tend to be preceded by a period of unhappiness and worry. Physical examinations had been given to 100 employees at an automobile factory six weeks before the plant closed and the men lost their jobs. Two years after they had been fired, the men were again given physical examinations. At this time there was a marked increase in the number of men suffering from hypertension, peptic ulcers, and arthritis. The magnitude of the increase in these illnesses could not be readily attributed to the mere passage of time, but could be caused by the worry associated with the loss of their jobs and efforts to find new work. Schmale (1958) subsequently found that thirty-one of forty-two patients newly admitted to a hospital had recently experienced events that gave rise to feelings of helplessness, hopelessness, and depression. Holmes and Masuda (1974) similarly demonstrated that individuals with many psychosocial problems in their lives are more prone to illness than individuals with fewer problems. All the stressful events experienced during an eighteen-month period were recorded and quantified, including such happenings as a death in the family or marital separation. The participants were seen again eight months later at which time they reported any illnesses they had experienced during that period. About half (49 percent) of those who had many stressful events in their lives reported illnesses, as compared to only 9 percent of those who had experienced few stressful events (Pelletier, 1977, p. 111).

Similar conclusions can be derived from research with other mammals. Working with a cancer-prone strain of rats, Riley (1975) placed a randomly selected half of the animals in highly stressful situations, while the others were provided with a peaceful life. Almost all (92 percent) of the stressed rats developed cancer as compared to only 7 percent of the peaceful (nonstressed) control group.

Returning to the human organism, there are many other studies indicative of stress effects. Russek (1965) reported that almost all (91 percent) of the hospitalized patients he interviewed soon after they had a heart attack mentioned negative factors in their lives that affected them not long before the infarction. These factors typically included strain on the job, problems at home, and general dissatisfaction and unhappiness. By contrast, only 20 percent of those in the control groups had such negative factors to mention. Similarly, Chambers and Reiser (1953) found that twenty-four of twenty-five patients hospitalized with congestive heart failure had had severe life problems immediately before they developed the disease. Common problems included death of or desertion by a spouse, sudden death of a child, rejection by an important person, and sudden loss of a love relationship. Comparable results were obtained by Medalie (cited by Theorell & Rahe, 1974) when he monitored the physical and mental health of a group of individuals over a five-year period. Those who had suffered a myocardial infarction during that period also were generally unhappier and had more dissatisfaction in their marriages. Wolf (1969) interviewed sixty-five individuals who had recently suffered a myocardial infarction and a like number of healthy controls. He then selected the ten most dissatisfied and depressed individuals and predicted that they would be the next ones to have additional heart attacks. All ten were among the first twenty-three who had a heart attack within a four-year followup period.

Another type of research design has been applied to the stress, unhappiness, and illness relationship. Heart functioning has been monitored by the electrocardiogram (EKG) while the experimenter talks to the participants. This has been done in two studies with healthy individuals (Sigler, 1967; Wolf, 1967), and also in a study with individuals who had cardiac problems (Stevenson, Dancan, Wolf, Ripley, & Wolff, 1949). Cardiac functioning became abnormal at those times when the experimenters talked to the participants about problems that frustrated or depressed them. The EKG showed premature ventricular contractions, atrial fibrillations, ventricular tachycardia, and other arrhythmias.

These studies and others reviewed by Lynch (1977) indicate that cardiac problems and other serious physical ailments appear to occur more often within a context of psychological stress and distress. Another series of investigations indicate that negative thoughts and emotions may be related to sudden death as well. Weisman and Hackett (1961) interviewed a series of hospitalized patients who had lost the will to live. As the authors stated, "Death held more appeal for these patients than did life." One patient, for example, saw death as a relief from all her torment and anguish, while another saw death as resolving all his problems and unhappiness. One looked forward to death because he expected to be reunited with his lost love. Some of these patients were not critically ill, and so there was no objective reason to expect that they would die—however, all did.

Engel (1971) reviewed a series of relatively young individuals who died suddenly and unexpectedly when they learned of the death of a person close to them. For instance, fourteen-year-old girl died upon learning of her brother's sudden death, and an eighteen-year-old died when she heard of her grandmother's death. Weisman and Hackett (1961) are among the clinicians who have observed that the attitudes of physically ill patients often seem predictive of their survival.

Studies of this kind indicate that negative thoughts and feelings can lead to illness and unexpected death. A related set of investigations will be reviewed next. These studies indicate that specific thoughts or beliefs can affect specific body functions. In other words, the belief that one has been exposed to poison ivy can produce the kind of skin reaction that follows actual contact with poison ivy. Taking an example from the other direction, the conviction that warts will go away can lead to their actual disappearance.

Effects of Specific Thoughts and Feelings

Ikemi and Nakagawa (1962) have demonstrated that some individuals who are sensitive to a plant of the poison ivy type in Japan show a complete skin reaction (itching, paupules, rash, blistering) when they *think* they have been exposed to the plant, but have actually had no such contact. They also demonstrated the reverse effect: some individuals who are sensitive to the plant do not show a skin reaction after actual exposure if they believe they are being exposed to something else (Barber, 1978).

The direct effects of thoughts and beliefs on bodily processes is also illustrated by the rather large number of studies indicating that warts are at times healed by direct suggestion (Barber, 1970, 1978; Johnson & Barber, 1978). Bloch (1927) long ago reported that a powerful suggestive procedure was effective in curing warts—in one session—in 31 percent of his patients (mostly children). This success rate is far above the expected base-rate of wart regression (Rulison, 1942). The successful outcome apparently was a result of the suggestive treatment procedure, one that is worth describing here. The warts were treated by a complex and impressive machine replete with flashing lights and noisy motors. The flashing lights and noisy motors were actually the only components of the machine that did anything. It was, in effect, a placebo machine. The patients were told that the machine would X-ray and kill the warts. After the procedure, the patients were told that the warts were now dead and should not be washed until they disappeared. Other investigators have since obtained similar results, even without a placebo machine. For instance, Allington (1934) found that thirty-five of eighty-four patients (42 percent were relieved of common warts after only one suggestive (placebo) treatment which consisted of intragluteal injection of distilled water given with the (mis)information that it was a potent wart remedy. As can be seen by the date of these studies, regressing warts by suggestive procedures is "old news" and is in the repertoire of a number of therapists today.

The effects of specific thoughts on specific bodily processes is also illustrated by four investigations involving a congenital skin disease (erythrodermia or ichtyosis), a condition that has no known etiology or successful treatment. Suggestive procedures have markedly relieved the disease in a number of instances. In the first of these studies, Mason (1952) was confronted with a sixteen-year-old patient whose skin (with the exception of face and chest) had been severely abnormal since birth. The skin was black, horny, covered with papillae, insensitive for several millimeters, and so hard and inelastic that it cracked and oozed blood-stained serum. Since there was no known effective treatment available for this disease, Mason tried suggestion. He first induced a relaxed, hypnotic state, and then suggested that the skin on his left arm would gradually become normal. Within a few days the hard skin on his left arm began to soften and change. Ten days later it was normal. In the same direct way, Mason suggested, session by session, that the back would heal . . . then the buttocks . . . the thighs, and so on. The skin continued to heal and returned to normal in accordance with the suggestions. This result commanded so much attention that three subsequent investigations were made (Kidd, 1966; Schneck, 1966; Wink, 1961). All showed that suggestions were, indeed, effective in ameliorating this congenital skin disease that had previously been viewed as untreatable.

The effects of thoughts and feelings on bodily processes are also illustrated by three more recent studies which showed that some women can enlarge their breasts by practicing the following simple regime at a certain time each day for about twelve weeks: (1) imagining that a sun lamp or hot towels on the breasts are making them pleasantly warm; (2) then suggesting to themselves that their breasts were tingling, becoming more sensitive, and growing (Staib & Logan, 1977; Willard, 1977; Williams, 1974). The typical woman participating in these studies showed an increase in breast circumference of about one and a half inches. Those who were best able to visualize the suggested changes showed the largest increases (Willard, 1977). When followed up over a three-month period, 81 percent of the enlargement in breast size was still present (Staib & Logan, 1977).

Finally, the effects of thoughts and feeling on the alteration of bodily functions is also illustrated by pseudocyesis (false pregnancy). This phenomenon is not as uncommon as one might suppose. Fried, Rakoff, Schopbach, and Kaplan (1951) reviewed 465 published cases of women who were not pregnant but believed they were. These women had either stopped or markedly reduced menstruation, showed weight gain, abdominal enlargement, and, in some cases, morning sickness, breast tenderness, and even "fetal" movements. A few went into so-called labor, but this condition ceased abruptly when the women were told they were not pregnant. In all these cases, the individual's body literally followed the contours of thought and expectation even though no physical cause was present.

TOWARD THE FUTURE

Who is the ideal healer? This question can now be answered, at least in its broad outlines. The most effective healers in the future will be those who combine the broad knowledge of physiological and pathological processes that we expect of a first-rate physician with the suggestive potency of the best hypnotist, and the love and compassion that has characterized the most successful religious, psychic, and spiritistic healers. Candidates for the healing professions will be selected for such personal qualities as love and compassion, as well as for suggestive potency and the superb scholarly abilities that are needed to assimilate the ever-increasing knowledge of the human organism in health and disease. Let us briefly consider what tomorrow's more effective healer will need from the realms of suggestive therapy, medicine, and healing.

Strengths and Limitations of Suggestive Therapy

Advances in knowledge have made it increasingly clear that health and illness are affected by our state of mind. Furthermore, verbal and nonverbal suggestions can have effects on our thoughts and feelings that either facilitate our recovery or confirm and intensify our disability. Reference has been made to only a few of the many studies and clinical reports which indicate that direct verbal suggestions can be therapeutic in the treatment of a wide variety of ailments. Despite the documented effectiveness of hypnosis or therapeutic suggestions, however, it is only the exceptional physician who employs such suggestions in a planful and systematic way. At least four factors have contributed to blocking the broader utilization of suggestions in medicine.

1. Medicine has had a strong organic bias during the past two or three centuries which allows little room for the possible effect of psychological factors. Often there has been discomfort and disdain when non-organic factors intrude because medicine has been keenly motivated to become scientific and disassociate itself from earlier practices.

2. Because of the dominance of the organic viewpoint, physicians have received little formal instruction on the potency of suggestive therapy. Very few physicians are aware, for example, that verbal suggestions can minimize the effects of burns (Chapman, Goodell, & Wolff, 1959; Delbouef, 1887; Ewin, 1979), alleviate "fish-skin" disease (congenital erythrodermia), cure congenital pachyonychia (Mullins, Murray & Shapiro, 1955), heal warts, both produce and alleviate cardiac arrythmias, reduce status asthmaticus, and, in brief, affect a wide variety of physiological systems and pathological manifestations (Barber, 1970, 1978; Bowers, 1979).

3. The relatively small number of physicians who are aware of the kinds of data cited in the preceding paragraph tend to misattribute the effects. It is commonly thought that such effects are brought about through hypnosis, by which is meant a rather mysterious state. Direct suggestion perhaps appears too simple, familiar, and obvious a technique, and more exotic explanations are sought.

Bernheim and others long ago found that the hypnotic state was not itself a crucial part of the process, and many studies subsequently have shown that suggestion, with or without hypnotic trance induction, is the effective process. This information is either not known to or has not registered upon many physicians. Most individuals respond to suggestions in the same way whether or not they have been exposed to a hypnotic induction procedure. A smaller number of people respond differentially to suggestions with and without hypnotic induction, but for some of them the effect of suggestions is actually greater *without* induction. How well individuals respond to suggestions does not depend upon formal rituals (hypnotic induction), although these rituals have become famous and, to some, beloved. The crucial variables include the individual's life history, relationship with the physician, attitudes, motivations, and expectancies toward the total situation, and the specific wording and implications of the suggestions (Barber, 1969, 1970; Barber, Spanos, & Chaves, 1974; Wilson & Barber, 1980).

4. Even when physicians are aware that their suggestions can be potent, they often do not know how to give these suggestions effectively. Suggestions are rarely effective when they are given in a rigid manner. They should be given in a natural manner within a caring relationship and worded specifically for this particular patient in this particular situation. Unfortunately, there are still few physicians (or other healers) who are able simultaneously to care deeply about the patient while giving direct verbal suggestions in a natural manner that is meaningful and acceptable to the patient.

In fact, whether or not verbal suggestions alter the patient's attitude, feelings, and emotions depends in part upon the characteristics of the person giving the suggestions. The therapist as a person is one of the most powerful variables in the situation. The patient will accept suggestions in a more profound way if the therapist is convinced of the truth of his or her statements, is highly regarded by the patient, and is not a cold, aloof individual but one who is caring, compassionate, loving.

There is an even more neglected aspect of formal training in suggestive therapy (or hypnotherapy, as it is more often presented). This is the tremendous potency and usefulness of suggestions given *nonverbally*. These suggestions occur continually whether or not they are recognized by the therapist. Implicit suggestions are deeply embedded in everything that any healer says, prescribes, or does. At the very minimum, the healer's actions as well as words convey the unspoken suggestion, "What I am doing will help you recover from your ailment." As Frank (1961, 1978) has pointed out, this implicit suggestion ("You will be healed") may be absolutely the most important factor in any approach to healing because it reduces anxiety about the illness.

Earlier in this chapter we cited data indicating that the history of medicine has been largely a history of nonverbal, suggestive (placebo) effects (Shapiro, 1971). Nonverbal suggestions were important in the healing temples of Isis, Serapis, or Aesculapius; in the charms, amulets, talismans, and herbs of ancient and medieval medicine; in the potions and drugs prescribed by physicians of the eighteenth and nineteenth centuries, and also in a very large number of effective remedies that were definitely not viewed as suggestive by either the laymen or physicians who used that at that time.

"Perkin's tractors" exemplify the suggestive techniques that were viewed by practically all involved as though potent organic remedies. Elisha Perkins, founder of the Connecticut Medical Society in 1796, became convinced that diseased tissues could be healed by metal. "Galvanism" was a newly discovered phenomenon at that time, and its potentials and limitations were anybody's guess. Perkins began using two pieces of metal in his medical practice. Each was about three inches long, one of iron, the other of copper. Perkins took care to patent his "tractors" which were moved lightly over the patient's diseased or painful areas. Many physicians had their set of tractors by the end of the eighteenth century, and about 5,000 documented cases proclaimed the remarkable healings they had produced. Many of these cures involved conditions that had been diagnosed as organic. Successes were reported with children and adults, and with animals as well (Dingwall, 1967). These cures were always attributed to the healing effects of the metals. Almost nobody seriously considered the possibility that the effective variable was actually the nonverbal suggestion that "this metal which I am moving over your diseased or painful area will heal you." But there was at least one questioning mind, and Haygarth (1801) in England carried out a series of experiments with nonpatented imitation tractors made of wood and other nonmetallic substances. He obtained his share of remarkable cures. His conclusion was that practically any nonmetallic object that was moved over the afflicted area could lead to relief *provided that the patients believed the objects to have curative properties.*

Suggestive factors (known in today's jargon as "placebo effects") play an important role in modern medicine and surgery. Beecher (1955, 1959) has summarized a mass of data on the effects of nondrugs (for example, a chemically inert capsule filled with salt water) on sick people. In all the studies he reviewed, the drug was no drug at all, but the recipient believed it to be a potent agent. In reviewing a set of five investigations, Beecher found that placebos produced satisfactory relief of severe post-operative pain in nearly one-third of 453 post-surgical patients. This finding becomes even more striking when we note that Lasagna and Beecher (1954) had also shown that a large dose of morphine relieved post-operative wound pain in only 75 percent of the patients. Beecher (1959) then showed that "of the average pain relief produced by a large dose of morphine in treating severe pain, nearly half must be attributed to a placebo (or suggestive effect)." He also reviewed data from ten investigations in which placebos were given to more than 600 patients for the relief of pain from angina pectoris, or alleviation of headache, seasickness, cough, the common cold, or anxiety and tension. In each study, the target symptoms was relieved by the placebo in at least 26 percent of the patients. On the average, the believed-in nondrug was effective in relieving the symptoms of about one-third of the patients.

Not only do placebos produce therapeutic results but they can also produce "toxic" effects. For instance, in one of his own investigations, Beecher (1955) found that 50 percent of the patients reported that a placebo made them feel drowsy. In another investigation 25 percent stated that a placebo had given them a headache, and 10 percent said it made them nauseated. Similarly, Wolf and Pinsky (1954) found that although most patients had only minor reactions to a placebo, three of their thirty-one patients had major reactions. Immediately upon taking the placebo, one patient had overwhelming weakness with palpitation and nausea. Soon after taking the placebo a second patient developed an itchy, erythematous, maculopapular rash, which was diagnosed by a dermatologist as dermatitis medicamentosa. The rash cleared quickly after the administration of placebos was stopped. Within ten minutes after taking placebo pills, a third patient had epigastric pains followed by watery diarrhea, urticaria, and angioneurotic edema of the lips. The same symptoms occurred two more times when she received the placebo pills. These and other data (Beecher, 1959) indicate that, at least in some patients, the mistaken belief that they have received a drug, along with their specific expectations from the drug, can lead to gross changes in their bodily functioning.

The power of suggestive effects has also been demonstrated many times in surgery. About thirty years ago, for example, a group of surgeons treated anginal pain by tying off the mammary artery in the chest with the purpose of increasing blood flow to the heart. This operation produced relief of anginal pain in 40 percent of the patients. In addition, those patients who were helped by the operation showed increased exercise tolerance and a significantly reduced need for their medication (nitroglycerin tablets). Subsequently, control operations were performed on a series of patients with angina. These patients believed they were receiving the same operation for angina (mammary artery ligation), but this did not happen. Instead, the skin was cut and stitches were made, but nothing more was done. The pseudo-operation was just as effective in relieving angina as the original operations in which the mammary arteries were ligated (Gross, 1966). The conclusion indicated by these findings was that the effective variable in relieving anginal pain was *not* the surgical operation per se but the implicit suggestion that accompanied the operation, namely: "This complex surgical operation which has helped so many others will also heal you."

Positive and Negative Aspects of Modern Medicine

The ideal future healer will be expert in the use of suggestive procedures, but will also have a thorough knowledge of medicine, including a firm grasp on the history of medicine and surgery. The healer will also have command of the spectrum of basic biological and medical sciences (anatomy, physiology, biochemistry, microbiology, pathology, and so on), and skill in applying these sciences to diagnosis and treatment.

Less obvious, perhaps, but also important will be the healer's familiarity with modern medicine's negative aspects. He will be intimately acquainted with the facts behind a conclusion such as the following: "Unfortunately, iatrogenic disease (disease produced by the doctor's treatment) can now take its place almost as an equal alongside the bacteria as an important factor in the pathogenesis of human illness" (Spain, 1963, quoted in Gross, 1966, p. 10). The well trained healer of the future will realize how many ailments of our time are the consequence of adverse reactions to prescribed drugs, to the prescription of inappropriate drugs, to overmedication, faulty blood transfusion, diagnostic accidents in biopsy, endoscopy, and many other procedures, infections from catheters, reactions to anesthetics, injection damage, overuse of x-rays, arteriograms, myelograms, and on and on (Barr, 1955; Gross, 1966; Illich, 1976; Mendelsohn, 1979; Schimmel, 1964). The ideal healer will be conversant with all the documentation which shows that drugs prescribed by physicians today may be doing almost as much harm as good. Furthermore, the healer will realize that some surgical procedures (as in many instances of tonsillectomies and hysterectomies) also do more harm than good.

Other pitfalls of modern medicine will also be avoided by this knowledgeable and dedicated healer. The patient will not be treated impersonally with unseasoned therapies and premature surgical procedures. The patient will not be locked into a totally passive role while in the hands of professionals. The patient will not be given a hasty diagnosis or misleading information (for instance, vague references to heart murmurs which can persuade healthy individuals to define themselves as sick, with unfortunate implications not only for this person but for others in his or her life.

This healer will not repeat the errors that many others continue to make, such as (1) failing to rely sufficiently on the body's own awesome healing processes, (2) intervening in complex and delicate bodily processes by prescribing unnecessary drugs with their surplus effects, (3) utilizing unnecessary radiological techniques, and (4) performing surgery on healthy tissues and organs. Stated otherwise, the ideal future healer will use drugs, X-rays, surgery, and other invasive procedures rarely and selectively. Much more often, these wise healers will rely on their uncontingent, unconditional love for the patient, on suggestive procedures, and on educational procedures. The latter include discussions of nutrition, interpersonal problems, or other difficulties which underlie or exacerbate the disorder. The healers will direct themselves to help the patient relax, become more serene, and be more able to flow with the events of his or her life, and thus to maximize the patient's own recuperative powers.

Using the Positive, Avoiding the Negative

Other things being equal, the deeper the healer's love for the patient, the more the patient is willing to accept the healer's verbal and nonverbal suggestions. These interrelated factors, however, can be separated at times. It appears that either love alone or suggestive potency alone is sufficient in helping some sick individuals recover.

Earlier in this chapter we summarized data indicating that the most important factor in healing is stimulating of the patient's own recuperative functions. These functions are enhanced to the extent that there is a reduction in fear, resentment, guilt, hopelessness, and other negative emotions. In turn, these "negative emotions" are reduced to the extent that the healer helps the patient feel "loved, lovable, and loving" (Bennett, 1980).

The history of hypnosis and suggestive therapeutics also shows that suggestions alone, without special love from the healer, are often sufficient to bring about recovery. Many hypnotists or suggestive therapists have been very loving people and close to their patients. But there is no doubt that some remarkable healings (for instance, the healing of warts by Johnson & Barber, 1978) were primarily the result of suggestions because the experimenter-hypnotist had to follow a standard protocol and relate to the client in a prescribed, formal way. There have been faith healers who were definitely shown to have no love for their patients and who nevertheless obtained cures apparently through suggestive effects alone. The well known healer Marjoe, for example, is credited with as many documented miraculous cures as any other person on the current scene. Yet Marjoe recently admitted in his post-retirement film autobiography that he did not care at all about his patients. Instead, his version of healing was a business in which he did his part (that is, calling upon Christ to heal the invalid) and received handsome fees for his services (Kruger, 1974, pp. 275-277).

As stated above, healers of the future will be trained broadly in the biomedical and psychological sciences after they have been selected for their ability to love others and for their suggestive potency. Effectiveness in administering verbal and nonverbal suggestions is related to many variables that need to be further investigated. These include high self-esteem on the part of the healer, loving willingness to give of oneself to the patient, and belief in the healing effectiveness of verbal suggestions, or in the effectiveness of nonverbal suggestive procedures such as laying-on-of-hands (Krieger, 1979). This is simply a starting list of variables that are likely to be important.

Since healers of the future will be thoroughly trained in the biomedical and psychological sciences, they will not be open to criticisms such as the following which have been leveled—with some justification—against some present-day lay healers:

1. Their limited understanding of the regenerative capacities of the human organism leads them to (mis)attribute the positive results to powers or forces within themselves. Among other disadvantages of this tendency is the development of personality and power cults around the healer which can have unfortunate results, as well as the unwitting self-deception involved in crediting one's own powers to the neglect of the patient's own contribution.

2. Their limited knowledge of physiology and pathology leads them to accept naive and mistaken diagnoses proferred by their patients, friends, or relatives.

3. Their ignorance of psychological dynamics in the etiology of disease leads them to claim unjustified miraculous healings of conditions they believe to be physical but which are actually of functional origin (conversion reactions and hysterical symptoms). Some forms of paralysis, blindness, deafness, and pain are among the conditions that often lead to these exaggerated claims.

4. Their unsophisticated readiness to declare that patients are cured leads some patients to avoid further treatment of life-threatening illnesses and thus may lead to premature death (Nolan, 1974).

Should we conclude, then, that the effectiveness of healing is drawn entirely from the known potencies of love and of verbal and nonverbal suggestions? This conclusion has the advantage of parsimony, although with a broad data base. Other possible factors, however, have not been ruled out. We need to look more closely at so-called psychic and spiritistic effects. There is no lack of anecdotal report in this area, but monumental research challenges remain to be surmounted. We are not in a position to accept or reject psychic and spiritistic claims at this time.

Curiosity demands further attention to factors involved in the effectiveness of healers such as Oskar Estebany who, among other feats, apparently has hastened wound healing in mice (Grad, Cadoret, & Paul, 1961). It is easy to assume that the recuperative powers of mice and other mammals cannot be affected by love and nonverbal suggestions from humans. This belief, however, may be erroneous. Mice and other mammals are very similar to us anatomically and physiologically. Furthermore, although other mammals differ from us in language functions, their feelings and emotions are much more similar to ours than is commonly supposed (Thorpe, 1974). Serious consideration should be given to the possibility that a human healer can affect the recuperative powers of other mammals in the same way that he would affect a human being who has never learned to speak, namely, by love and nonverbal suggestions transmitting a sense of caring and security. This possibility could be tested empirically by inviting Estebany (or other healers) to heal mice or other mammals when they are aware and when they are not aware of his presence and healing actions. Further research is also needed to replicate and extend recent studies which indicated that Estebany and possibly other lay healers can affect plants, human hemoglobin, and the human enzyme, trypsin (Grad, 1964, 1967; Krieger, 1979; Miller, 1972; Smith, 1973).

Understanding precisely what the healer does and does not do, and how far these processes might extend, is an aim that is still well beyond the reach of current data and perhaps current methodology as well. Enough has been learned, however, clearly to locate much of the magic in the love, compassion, and suggestive skills of the healer and the recuperative powers of the patient's body when sparked by belief and liberated from anxiety and dread.

HEALING THE AGED?

This chapter has explored three traditions that have sought to bring relief and facilitate recuperation to the sick and disabled. No specific reference has been made to the aged person. Do any or all of these traditions have anything to offer to the man or woman whose problems appear to be mandated by time rather than by unfortunate happenstance? Once healed, the young person may go on to enjoy many years of excellent health and well-being. Is healing truly possible with those who, already afflicted with age-related disorders, will surely continue to age and die?

Therapy with the aged raises questions of value and philosophy as well as technique. Pragmatic and theoretical issues related to therapy of the ill, impaired, vulnerable aged will be examined in the next chapter.

REFERENCES

Allington, H.V. Sulpharsphenamine in the treatment of warts. *Archives of Dermatology and Syphilology*, 1934, *29*, 687–690.

Atkinson, D.T. *Magic, myth, and medicine.* New York: World Publishing Company, 1956.

Barber, T.X. *Hypnosis: a scientific approach.* New York: Van Nostrand Reinhard, 1969.

Barber, T.X. *LSD, marihuana, yoga, and hypnosis.* Hawthorne, N.Y.: Aldine Publishing Co., 1970.

Barber, T.X. Hypnosis, suggestions, and psychosomatic phenomena: A new look from the standpoint of recent experimental studies. *American Journal of Clinical Hypnosis*, 1978, *21*, 13–27.

Barber, T.X., Spanos, N.P., & Chaves, J.F. *Hypnosis, imagination, and human potentialities.* Elmsford, N.Y.: Pergamon, 1974.

Barr, D.P. Hazards of modern diagnosis and therapy—the price we pay. *Journal of the American Medical Association*, December 10, 1955, pp. 1452–1456.

Bauer, J. Sudden unexpected death. *Postgraduate Medicine*, 1957, *22*, 34–45.

Bean, W.B. The natural history of error (surgical error: lo the poor tonsils!). *Transactions of the Association of American Physicians*, 1959, *22*, 40–55.

Bennet, A. Personal communication, September 16, 1980, Department of Psychology, Boston College, Chestnut Hill, Mass.

Bloch, B. Ueber die Heilung der Warzen durch suggestion. *Klinische Wochenschrift*, 1927, *6*, 2272–2275; 2320–2325.

Bowers, K.S., & Kelly, P. Stress, disease, psychotherapy, and hypnosis. *Journal of Abnormal Psychology*, 1979, *88*, 490–505.

Caton, R. *The temples and ritual of Asklepios.* London: C.J. Clay & Sons, 1900.

Chambers, W.N., & Reiser, M.F. Emotional stress in the precipitation of congestive heart failure. *Psychosomatic Medicine*, 1953, *15*, 38–60.

Deleuze, J.P.F. Rules of magnetizing (1825). In R.E. Shor & M.T. Orne (Eds.), *The nature of hypnosis.* New York: Holt, Rinehart & Winston, 1966.

Dingwall, E.J. *Abnormal hypnotic phenomena: A survey of nineteenth-century cases* (Vol. I: France). New York: Barnes & Noble, 1967.

Doyle, J.C. Unnecessary hysterectomies: Study of 6, 242 operations in thirty hospitals during 1948. *Journal of the American Medical Association*, January 31, 1953, pp. 360-365.

Edelstein, E.J., & Edelstein, L. *Ascelpius* (2 vols.). Baltimore: Johns Hopkins Press, 1945.

Editorial: Tonsillectomy and adenoidectomy. *Canadian Medical Association Journal*, December 28, 1963, pp. 1334-1335.

Ellenberger, H.G. Mesmer and Puysegur: From magnetism to hypnotism. *Psychoanalytic Review*, 1965, *52*, 137-153.

Emerson, R.W. *The portable Emerson.* New York: Viking, 1965.

Engel, G.L. Sudden and rapid death during psychological stress: Folklore or folk wisdom? *Annals of Internal Medicine*, 1971, *74*, 771-782.

Ewin, D.B. Hypnosis in burn therapy. In G.D. Burrows, D.R. Collison, & L. Dennerstein (Eds.), *Hypnosis 1979.* New Uprl: Elsevier/North Holland Biomedical Press, 1979.

Frank, J.D. *Persuasion and healing.* Baltimore: Johns Hopkins Press, 1961.

Frank, J.D. Psychotherapy and the healing arts. In J.L. Fosshage & P. Olsen (Eds.), *Healing: Implications for psychotherapy.* New York: Human Sciences Press, 1978.

Fried, P.H., Rakoff, A.E., Schopbach, R.R., & Kaplan, A.J. Pseudocyesis: A psychosomatic study in gynecology. *Journal of the American Medical Association*, 1951, *145*, 1329-1335.

Fromm, E. *The art of loving.* New York: Harper, 1956.

Glaser, R.J. *The body is the hero.* New York: Random House, 1976.

Goddard, H.H. The effects of mind on body as evidence by faith cures. *American Journal of Psychology*, 1899, *10*, 431-502.

Grad, B. A telekinetic effect on plant growth. *International Journal of Parapsychology*, 1964, *6*, 473.

Grad, B. The 'laying on of hands': Implications for psychotherapy, gentling, and the placebo effect. *Journal of the American Society for Psychical Research*, 1967, *61*, 286-305.

Grad, B., Cadoret, R.J., & Paul, G.I. The influence of an unorthodox method of treatment on wound healing of mice. *International Journal of Parapsychology*, 1961, *3*, 5-24.

Gross, M.L. *The doctors.* New York: Random House, 1966.

Guthrie, D.J., Underwood, E.A., Thomson, W.A.R., & Richardson, R.G. History of medicine. *Encylopedia Britannica* (15th ed.). Chicago: Encyclopedia Britannica, Inc., 1977 (Vol. 11).

Hartland, J. *Medical and dental hypnosis and its clinical applications.* Baltimore: Williams & Williams, 1966.

Holmes, T.H., & Masuda, G. Life changes and illness susceptibility. In B.S. Doboswend & B.P. Doboswend (Eds.), *Stressful Life Events.* N.Y.: Wiley, 1974, pp. 45-72.

Ikemi, Y., & Nakagawa, S.   A psychosomatic study of contagious dermatitis. *Kyushu Journal of Medical Science*, 1962, *13*, 335–350.

Illich, I. *Medical nemesis.* New York: Random House, 1976.

Johnson, R.F.Q., & Barber, T.X. Hypnosis, suggestions, and warts: An experimental investigation implicating the importance of "believed-in efficacy." *American Journal of Clinical Hypnosis*, 1978, *20*, 165–174.

Kasl, S.V., & Cobb, S. Blood pressure changes in men undergoing job loss: A preliminary report. *Psychosomatic Medicine*, 1970, *32*, 19–38.

Kidd, C.B. Congenital icrhyosiform erythrodermia treated by hypnosis. *British Journal of Dermatology*, 1966, *78*, 101–105.

Kilpatrick, G.S. Observer error in medicine. *Journal of Medical Education*, 1963, *38*(1), 38–42.

Krieger, D. *The therapeutic touch: How to use your hands to help or to heal.* Englewood Cliffs, N.J.: Prentice–Hall, 1979.

Krippner, S., & Villoldo, A. *The realms of healing.* Millbrae, Calif.: Celestial Arts, 1976.

Kroger, W.S. *Clinical and experimental hypnosis.* Philadelphia: J.B. Lippincott, 1977.

Korger, W.S., & Fezler, W.D. *Hypnosis and behavior modification: Imagery conditioning.* Philadelphia: J.B. Lippincott, 1976.

Kruger, H. *Other healers, other cures: A guide to alternative medicine.* Indianapolis: Bobbs–Merrill, 1974.

LaPatra, H. *Healing: The coming revolution in holistic medicine.* New York: McGraw–Hill, 1978.

LeShan, L. *The medium, the mystic, and the physicist.* New York: Viking, 1974.

Ludwig, A.M. An historical survey of the early routes of Mesmerism. *International Journal of Clinical and Experimental Hypnosis*, 1964, *12*, 205–217.

Lynch, J.J. *The broken heart: The medical consequences of loneliness.* New York: Basic Books, 1977.

MacHovec, F.J. Hypnosis before Mesmer. *American Journal of Clinical Hypnosis*, 1979, *22*, 85–90.

Mason, A.A. Ichthyosis and hypnosis. *British Medical Journal*, 1955, *2*, 57.

Meares, A. *A system of medical hypnosis.* Philadelphia: Saunders, 1960.

Meek, G.W. *Healers and the healing process.* Wheaton, Ill.: Theosophical Publishing House, 1977.

Mendelsohn, R.S. *Confessions of a Medical Heretic.* N.Y.: Warner Books, 1979.

Miller, R.N. The positive effect of prayer on plants. *Psychic Magazine*, April 1972, p. 25.

Muller, J. *Handbuch der Physiologie des Menschen.* Coblenz: Vostrag, 1834–1840.

Mullins, J.F., Murray, N., & Shapiro, E.M. Pachyonchia congenia: A review and a new approach to treatment. *Archives of Dermatology and Syphilology*, 1955, *71*, 265–268.

Nolen, W.A. *Healing: A doctor in search of a miracle.* New York: Random House, 1974.

Pattison, E.M., Lapins, N.A., & Doerr, H.A. Faith healing: A study of personality and function. *Journal of Nervous and Mental Disease*, 1973, *157*, 397–409.

Pelletier, K.R. *Mind as healer, mind as slayer.* New York: Delta, 1977.

Riley, V. Mouse mammary tumors: Alteration of incidence as apparent function of stress. *Science*, 1975, *189*, 465–467;

Rogers, M.P., Dubey, D., & Reich, P. The influence of the psyche and the brain on immunity and disease susceptibility: A critical review. *Psychosomatic Medicine*, 1979, *41*, 147–164.

Rossman, P.L. Organic diseases simulating functional disorders. *General Practitioner*, August 1973, pp. 78–83.

Rulison, R.H. Warts: A statistical study of 921 cases. *Archives of Dermatology and Syphilogy*, 1942, *46*, 62–74.

Russek, H.I. Stress, tobacco, and coronary heart disease in North American professional groups. *Journal of the American Medical Association*, 1965, *192*, 189–194.

Sanders, B.S. Completeness and reliability of diagnoses in therapeutic practice. Paper presented at annual meeting of the American Public Health Association (Statistics Section), November 1963.

Sanford, A. *The healing light.* (Rev. ed.). Plainfield, N.J.: Logus International, 1972.

Schimmel, E.M. The hazards of hospitalization. *Annals of Internal Medicine*, January 1964, pp. 100–110.

Schleiffer, S.J., Keller, S.E., & McKegney, F.P. Bereavement and lymphocyte function. Paper presented at annual meeting of American Psychiatric Association, San Francisco, May 1980.

Schmale, A.H., Jr. Relationship of separation and depression to disease: I. A report on a hospitalized medical population. *Psychosomatic Medicine*, 1958, *20*, 259–277.

Schneck, J.M. *The principles and practice of hypnoanalysis.* Springfield, Ill.: Charles C. Thomas, 1965.

Schneck, J.M. Hypnotherapy for iichthyosis. *Psychosomatics*, 1966, *1*, 233–235.

Shapiro, A.K. Placebo effects in medicine, psychotherapy, and psychoanalysis. In A.E. Bergin & S.L. Garfield (Eds.), *Handbook of psychotherapy and behavior change: An empirical analysis.* New York: John Wiley, 1971.

Shealy, C.N. *Occult medicine can save your life.* New York: Dial Press, 1975.

Shor, R.E. The fundamental problem in hypnosis research as viewed from historic perspective. In E. Fromm & R.E. Shor (Eds.), *Hypnosis: Developments in research and new perspectives.* (2nd ed.). Hawthorne, N.Y.: Aldine Publishing Co., 1979.

Sigler, L.H. Emotion and atherosclerotic heart disease. I: Electrocardiographic changes observed in the recall of past emotional disturbance. *British Journal of Medical Psychology*, 1967, *40*, 55.

Smith, M.J. The influence on enzyme growth by the 'laying on of hands'. In *Dimensions of healing*. Los Altos, Calif.: Academy of Parapsychology and Medicine, 1973.

Sorokin, P.T. *The ways and power of love*. Boston: Beacon Press, 1954.

Spain, D.M. *The complications of modern medical practice*. New York: Grune & Stratton, 1963.

Staib, A.R., & Logan, D.R. Hypnotic stimulation of breast growth. *American Journal of Clinical Hypnosis*, 1977, *19*, 201–208.

Stevenson, I., Dancan, J., Wolf, S., Ripley, A., & Wolff, H.G. Life situations, emotions, and extrasystoles. *Psychosomatic Medicine*, 1949, *11*, 257–266.

Theorell, T., & Gahe, R.H. Psychosocial characteristics of subjects with myocardial infarction in Stockholm. In E.K. Gunderson & R.H. Rahe (Eds.), *Life stress and illness*. Springfield, Ill.: Charles C. Thomas, 1974.

Thorpe, W.H. *Animal nature and human nature*. New York: Doubleday, 1974.

Weatherhead, L.D. *Psychology, religion and healing*. (Rev. ed.). Nashville, Tenn.: Abingdon Press, 1952.

Weisman, A.D., & Hackett, T.P. Predilection to death: Death and dying as a psychiatric problem. *Psychosomatic Medicine*, 1961, *23*, 232–251.

Wetterstrand, O.G. *Hypnotism and its applications in practical medicine*. Vienna: Urban & Schwarzenberg, 1891.

Willard, R.D. Breast enlargement through visual imagery and hypnosis. *American Journal of Clinical Hypnosis*, 1977, *19*, 195–200.

Williams, J.E. Stimulation of breast growth by hypnosis. *Journal of Sex Research*, 1974, *10*, 316–326.

Wilson, S.C., & Barber, T.X. Vivid fantasy and hallucinatory abilities in the life histories of excellent hypnotic subjects ("somnambules"): Preliminary report with female subjects. Paper presented at annual meeting of the American Association for the Study of Mental Imagery, Minneapolis, June 1980.

Wink, C.A.S. Congenital ichthyosiform erthrodermia treated by hypnosis: Report of two cases. *British Medical Journal*, 1961, *2*, 741–743.

Wolf, S. The end of the rope: The role of the brain in cardiac death. *Canadian Medical Association Journal*, 1967, *97*, 1022–1024.

Wolf, S. Psychosocial forces in myocardial infarction and sudden death. *Circulation*, 1969, *40* (Suppl. IV), 74–81.

Wolf, S., & Wolff, H.G. *Human gastric function*. New York: Oxford University Press, 1947.

2 THERAPY BEGINS

LIFE IN A GERIATRIC HOSPITAL

Cushing Hospital is in some ways an unique and in other ways a typical institution for the aged. It is typical in the sense that the residents include many people who have lost functional abilities and sources of satisfaction that sustained them earlier in life. Most obvious, perhaps, is their loss of physical function. Some men and women require assistance with virtually every activity of daily life. Others have marked limitations in strength, mobility, and range of motion. Unfortunately, there seems to be no limit on the number of illnesses and debilitating conditions that can afflict the same individual. Here is a woman with diabetes, arthritis, and a heart condition. There is a man who has become blind and nearly deaf, and is also prone to kidney and bladder infections. Furthermore, the diagnosis "organic brain syndrome" is a common one. Problems in attention, concentration, memory, and what Raymond B. Cattell (1968) has described as "fluid intelligence" abound.

The combinations of disability are sometimes especially cruel. A mentally intact octogenarian may be almost entirely immobile and dependent on others for care and stimulation, while another person of the same age retains much physical independence but wanders about in a confused, disoriented state. Additionally, the mix of residents is quite pronounced. Some people have scarcely had a sick day in their lives until a trauma (for example, a stroke or a fall resulting in a broken hip) disrupted their continuity. Others have lived in the community all of their lives, but eventually declined to the point where neither the family (if available) nor other support systems could meet their needs. Still others have had troubled existences all along, living in and out of mental hospitals. In fact, some have been more "in" than "out," and have arrived finally at a geriatric hospital because their current problems were more those of a frail and vulnerable old person than of a psychiatric patient. The population of Cushing Hospital also includes some men and women who spent much of their childhood and adult years in a facility for the mentally retarded. Most of these "types" (a term that we use reluctantly because each person is primarily an individual) are familiar in other facilities for the aged across the nation. And each type has its own distinctive profile of sorrow, even tragedy. Among the mentally retarded residents of Cushing Hospital, for example, are men and women who might well have lived happily in the community all their lives if they had received appropriate services instead of being merely "warehoused" for so many years. (These people, by the way, almost without exception, have adjusted very well to the open and relatively enriched environment of Cushing Hospital.)

After having said all this, we have barely touched upon the problems that weigh most heavily on old people who live in institutions. Everybody knows the words, and almost everybody knows the experiences. Who of us has not been lonely? Who has not felt isolated, even abandoned? Who has not sunk into a mood of regret, bitterness, or self-recrimination about the past? Who has not felt anxious about the threats and demands of the moment? And who has not despaired for the future? These are all experiences that belong to the human condition in general, not just to the institutionalized aged. But an institution is a place where such negative emotional states—and more—are concentrated, and where one person's misery is apt to add to another's.

It is almost a law of nature. Gather together hundreds of people, both old and sick, who recognize that they have been ejected from the community, even if for "their own good." Place the facility itself at the bottom of almost every decisionmaker's priority list. Compete for staff with more glamorous components of the health-care delivery system. Require compliance with every conceivable policy and regulation, but offer little practical assistance, and seldom express appreciation for a job well done. The predictable result is misery generating misery—for staff as well as residents.

The situation described up to this point is more or less applicable to many facilities that are devoted to the care of the multiply-impaired aged. Yet the reality is sometimes more positive than all these negative elements would seem to imply. There are redeeming features. In the most neglected facilities we can find staff whose personal compassion and good nature transcend circumstances. Supportive relationships develop. People find ways to make life more tolerable. In the more self-respecting facilities, there is even more support, and life is a little more tolerable. However,—and this is an important point—seldom is the facility organized around or dedicated to the support of its residents as distinct and individual persons. Good things sometimes happen despite all the limitations and problems. We thought it was time to create a situation in which developing the good things was the essential aim.

CUSHING HOSPITAL: BEFORE HOLISTIC THERAPY

What we have been working toward at Cushing Hospital is of more than local interest because, as already noted, our circumstances in many respects resemble those of other facilities for the aged across the land. If the holistic therapy program has some value, then, this value is within reach of other health-care providers as well.

The distinctive configuration of advantages, disadvantages, and just plain oddities that comprise Cushing Hospital include the following:

1. By Massachusetts law, Cushing is a general hospital, yet it serves only the aged.

2. It is operated through the Commonwealth of Massachusetts' Executive Office of Human Services, under the specific responsibility of the Department of Mental Health—yet it is not a mental hospital. (All admissions are voluntary; there are no locked wards or rooms, and so on.) This administrative setup is something of a historical accident, but it has seemed to work and, despite continued discussion and weighing of alternatives, with DMH it remains.

3. The physical facility was constructed to serve the needs of the armed forces of the United States near the end of World War II. With this purpose in mind, the hospital was built to accommodate more than 1,700 short-term patients. The single-story construction on an attractive campus remains an advantage. The place was not built for privacy or geriatric care, nor for its own longevity. After a brief period of use by the Veterans Administration, it was transferred to the Commonwealth of Massachusetts where it started business as perhaps the nation's first all-geriatric hospital, most likely at least the first operated by the state government. The buildings have been maintained vigilantly and remain serviceable, although they cry out louder and louder for replacement.

4. The strength of the hospital is two-fold: a staff with more competence and compassion than money can buy, and a steady core of support from neighboring communities. Cushing never became a refuge for incompetent professionals, nor was it a forbidding fortress on the hill. Neighborhood children bike through the campus, joggers jog, and the little guard station by the gate has been reduced to the status of a relic.

5. Professional services at Cushing were exceptional in the facility's early days. There were not many other institutions a quarter of a century ago where geriatric patients could receive not only medical care from a staff of full-time house physicians and state-of-the-art nursing care but also dental care, occupational therapy, physical therapy, recreation therapy, rehabilitation team therapy, and advocacy, counseling, and assessment from the social service and psychology departments. A community itself, as well as a hospital, Cushing also had many support services such as dietary, housekeeping, engineering, and security (including a fire department). Consultants came in regularly to bring their specialty skills, and a volunteer service was working hard to foster community involvement. A library for the residents (as distinct from a small but well furbished professional library), a barbershop and beauty parlor, and a canteen were among the other amenities. Staff members worked on their own time to rehabilitate the swimming pool and greenhouse left behind by the federal occupants, and these, too, became part of the life-supportive activities. Cushing became known for a number of its contributions to the field, including the first systematic study of dying and death among the aged (for example, Weisman & Kastenbaum, 1968), and

its pioneering role in using and evaluating moderate alcohol beverage service with the aged (for example, Kastenbaum, 1972; Mishara & Kastenbaum, 1980). The place was humming!

6. For another decade, Cushing maintained its standard of quality care, but there was little in the way of new developments. In the meantime, interest in aging had risen across the country. Soon there were administrators with both knowledge and commitment to better geriatric care, supported by growing expertise in the emerging field of gerontology. Much of what had been distinctive and valuable at CH could now also be found at other facilities with a commitment to quality, and additional programs and services were also introduced. There was by now a definite dichotomy between high and low quality institutions for the aged. It had been shown that many professional services not only could be offered to the institutionalized aged but could have effective results. Some health-care providers took advantage of this knowledge; others, to this day, act as though no program is a good program.

The situation had changed again by the time we were ready to begin the holistic therapy program. Some of the change was for the worse. As people in the health-care professions well know, there is a nationwide shortage of nurses. This is a story in itself, but the relevant point here is that hospitals in general are having difficulty in attracting registered nurses. The attraction of hospital work seems to have diminished for other people as well. Good attendants have been increasingly hard to find. Furthermore, many of the staff who had given years of service to Cushing were now reaching retirement age, and some felt worn out. New people could be attracted in the allied health fields, but Cushing, along with many other facilities, has had to struggle more than ever to provide adequate coverage on a twenty-four-hour, seven-day-a-week basis. This tiresome recital of staffing problems is more relevant than we would wish it to be. A hospital is something of a living organism, and the status of its own holistic health and vigor at any point in time must be considered. We would be starting the holistic therapy program, then, at a time when the all-important nursing staff felt "straight-out" in their efforts to maintain quality care, their energies extended and their own peace of mind disturbed by the everyday demands they worked so hard to meet.

The nurses were not asking for a new therapeutic program. They were asking for more nurses—a reasonable request. A new program, in fact, could hardly help but be perceived as an extra burden and perhaps a distraction as well. Nevertheless, the new program was introduced. At the same time, renewed efforts were made to recruit more high quality nursing staff, and to provide more satisfactions and enriching experiences for those who were still with us. Although these programs are relevant to the whole picture, they will not be discussed here.

We also slowed the flow of new admissions. This decision was difficult. Many sick and vulnerable aged in the community seek admission to Cushing, and for some there are few satisfactory alternatives. We did not want to lower the standards of care, however, and felt it necessary to lessen the burden on the nursing staff and other direct care personnel. Over a period of time, the census was reduced from the 505 who were there the day the first member of this team (R.K.) arrived, to about 430, a level that has since remained fairly stable. Other positive changes were made, including the expansion of the recreation therapy service to reach more residents who were ward-bound and could seldom come to the Captain's Chair (the center of recreational activities which resembles a comfortable neighborhood pub). Expressive therapy was introduced, and arrangements made to have some program people available on evenings and weekends. The Cushing Hospital auxiliary also gained a second wind and soon built itself up to an all-time peak in membership, providing a variety of services and resources useful to the residents.

Still, when the new superintendent (R.K.) had become not quite so new, it was apparent to him that loneliness, anxiety, and despair had not been banished. There were programs of many kinds, but obviously something was missing. It was felt that these men and women, averaging more than eighty years of age and likely to end their lives at Cushing, required and deserved a sustaining relationship. Every resident should be an important and distinctive individual to at least one other person. We could not count upon the direct-care staff to assume this responsibility because they already had specific tasks they could not lay aside. Although they provided comfort and affection as best they could, they seldom had the opportunity to cultivate and maintain the type of core relationship that seemed necessary. It also seemed important that the helping person be somebody who is free from specific instrumental tasks. The relationship itself would be what mattered most. Theoretically, social workers and psychologists already on the staff might have taken part in the new program. In practice, however, their numbers were few, and they had already taken on other responsibilities that were not easily relinquished. The new program would have to begin with new people.

A Special Projects Division was established. The holistic therapy program emerged as one of its activities, the only one to be discussed here. Joining Cushing as director of SPD was Theodore X. Barber. Sheryl C. Wilson became the next member of this staff and provided much of the clinical supervision for the therapists. Beverly L. Ryder and Lisa B. Hathaway were the first therapists in this program, selected for their personal qualities as caring people. Judy Doran and Andrea George joined the SPD staff later and, more recently, Linda Enos. (Most of the case histories in this book come from the work of Ryder and Hathaway; some early experiences of Doran and George are also included.) Robert Johnson has provided specialized supervision and also shared with Barber the responsibility for communicating the therapeutic goals and techniques to the hospital staff at large.

PHILOSOPHY AND APPROACH

Our conception of the program flows in part from the material presented in our analysis of the interweaving histories of medicine, suggestive therapy, and healing. Positive suggestion and the expectation of helping and being helped obviously would be important. The concept of *healing* was also salient in our minds, but we recognized that this term means many things to many people. We shared a general view of the human organism as a resourceful, self-repairing, self-correcting agent. Centuries of healing and therapeutic efforts seem to be finding confirmation and more precise explanation through modern science, especially the realm that has been known by some as psychosomatic medicine (a dubious term, but it gets the point across). We believed that even people who suffer from multiple impairments retain some ability to spark their own recovery or compensate adequately. It seemed reasonable to offer these people a special kind of relationship, a relationship intended to help them realize their own potentials for overcoming disability and distress.

We wanted our own expectations to be reasonable. The realities of advanced age and multiple impairment (including impairments in the sensory and cognitive processes that are important in therapy) stood before us. Unlike the papyrus written in 1600 B.C., we did not propose to "transform an old man into a youth of twenty." And yet, neither ourselves nor anybody else could say with assurance what might be the outer limits for progress. We did think that our interpersonal intervention might help some patients in their physical as well as mental and emotional status. As a matter of fact, it would be hard to imagine either a physical or a psychological intervention that would not affect the whole person. We recognized that we would learn the potentials and limits only by trying. Cautiously, then, we permitted the term *healing* to remain within our repertoire.

The recent work of Dolores Krieger (cited earlier) provided one link with efforts other than our own. Krieger and her nursing colleagues are among those who have emphasized the value of touch and intimacy in treatment. This represents a revival or bringing-forward of a long tradition of therapeutic touch. Some practitioners see little difference between touch that is intended to be therapeutic, and touch that is healing. We do not have to resolve this problem immediately. The most relevant point is that gentle touching appeared to be an appropriate dimension of the therapeutic program we were in the process of developing.

The program was also designed with experience from geriatrics and gerontology in mind. A review of the clinical and social literature suggests that many old people—not only those who are institutionalized—are deprived of touch and intimate human contact. When we speak of a person "losing touch with reality," we are indeed speaking in earnest. The isolated old person (in community or institution) has, to some extent, lost touch with the human race. Furthermore, characteristic changes with age include a reduction of sensitivity across the sensory modes, another factor that tends to leave the individual with a more depleted stimulus field. Touch, therefore, seemed to be one direct and sensible way of restoring contact.

Until recent years there had been an infamous neglect of psychotherapy with the aged (for example, Kastenbaum, 1963). Fortunately, this situation has started to improve (for example, Storandt, Siegler, & Elias, 1978). We judged that some of the Cushing residents could benefit from more conventional forms of therapy, but that these people were definitely in the minority. The therapy we envisioned might have the effect of helping people reach a level at which other treatment modalities could become appropriate. This would parallel what we hoped to accomplish on the physical side: as people started feeling better about themselves and took more interest in their own recovery, all the other types of care being offered (medical, nursing, physical therapy, and so on) might then become more effective.

It might be interesting to mention a possible type of therapeutic approach that we decided *not* to include in this program, namely, behavior modification. Behavior modification is an approach that some of the present writers have used in other situations, including the geriatric. Our exclusion of this approach here does not represent opposition or lack of appreciation for what can be accomplished with a well conceived, well executed behavior modification program, nor does it blind us to the many happenings that could be interpreted in terms of various reinforcement theories. Our intent instead was to offer a relationship that was spectacularly *non* contingent. The old men and women would be accepted, valued, and cherished no matter what. This approach and behavior modification would have a hard time living side by side. One of the authors (S.C.W.) later described this facet of the program as "unconditional love therapy." It is an odd phrase to twentieth century ears, but it is accurate.

We did need a *name* for the kind of therapy that was to be offered. Many name-candidates came forth, and some of them had their trial periods. *Healing* expressed something of our aim, but as time went on we were less comfortable with this term. It was clear that the therapists were doing many other things besides those involved in the usual descriptions of healing. Furthermore, we were reluctant to cloak ourselves in a term that had so many surplus and ambiguous meanings. To this day, we do not have complete agreement on a name. The hospital staff in general has come to our rescue with the designation of *one-to-one therapy*. It is now routine for other services to refer residents for one-to-one therapy. Although this term will do for an in-house designation, by that slight privilege which comes to the author whose fingers tap out the final manuscript, when we need a name for this approach, it will be *holistic therapy* until a better term comes along. Drawbacks this term has. But it also tells us clearly that we are concerned with helping the *person* more than in tinkering with any of the components and dimensions of the person, and that such an approach must also recognize and release the life-giving potentials of the environment as well.

REFERENCES

Cattell, R.B.   Are I.Q. tests intelligent? *Psychology Today*, 1968, *1*, 56-62.

Kastenbaum, R.   The reluctant therapist. *Geriatrics*, 1963, *18*, 296-301.

Kastenbaum, R.   Beer, wine, and mutual gratification in the gerontopolis. In D.P. Kent, R. Kastenbaum, & S.S. Sherwood, (Eds.), *Research, planning, and action for the elderly.* New York: Behavioral Publications, 1972.

Mishara, B.L., & Kastenbaum, R.   *Alcohol and old age.* New York: Grune & Stratton, 1980.

Storandt, M., Siegler, I.C., & Elias, M.F. (Eds.) *The clinical psychology of aging.* New York: Plenum Press, 1978.

Weisman, A.D., & Kastenbaum, R.   *The psychological autopsy: A study of the terminal phase of life.* New York: Behavioral Publications, 1968.

3 HOLISTIC THERAPY

This chapter and the next comprise the heart of the book. The rest is commentary. A few things need to be said about the purposes this section is intended to serve and the manner of presentation.

Generalities have their place, but access to process and detail is essential for the understanding of any human interaction. You could form a more adequate impression of a holistic therapy sequence if you donned a *Tarnkappe* and witnessed the proceedings without influencing them. Cloaks of invisibility, however, seem to have disappeared from the shelf by Charlemagne's time. In our own time, the detailed case history appears the most sensible approach. The reader can either become a quasi-participant through imaginative involvement, or maintain a hawk-eyed distance. The interactions can be carved up with surgical gusto, or comprehended as a Gestalt — developing, fluctuating, and shimmering through time. Whatever the reader's aims and style, the case history seems to offer the most natural and effective way to share holistic therapy with geriatric patients.

But how should the case histories themselves be presented? There are several possibilities, all with their advantages and disadvantages. We have selected a single and consistent focus: what the therapist has done and experienced from the therapist's own view. In making this decision we reasoned that it would provide the most intimate and life-like perspective. It would also make it possible for both the reader and the authors to examine the process in detail. This approach has its virtues and vices from a methodological standpoint. We happen to think at this stage of our knowledge and craft, it is the approach we can all learn from most fully.

The case-presentation method *is* a method, if a simple one. This is how we went about it:

1.   The therapists met regularly with one of the authors (R.K.). These were reporting, not supervisory, sessions per se, although on occasion the boundaries were blurred. The proceedings were taped and subsequently transcribed.

2.   The sessions usually focused on the therapist's work with one particular Cushing Hospital patient. There were occasional variations, for instance, one or more therapists discussing a problem or phenomenon that had come up in a number of cases. The case-history section here draws entirely from the single-case presentations; some of the material from other sessions is taken into account in the commentary chapters.

3.   The designated listener attempted to serve as a stand-in for the reader. This meant that there would be questions to clarify what had been said (and translating facial expressions and gestures to the verbal medium). There would also be questions of a more probing sort, some of them aptly classified as *advocatus diaboli.* The listener assumed that the reader would have some critical questions along the way just as, indeed, the listener himself did. In general, the questions were intended to help the therapist convey as clearly as possible what she did, why she did it, what effects, if any, followed, and how she felt during the process. Additionally, some attempt was made to develop a situational context for the therapeutic process.

4.   The transcripts were edited with certain guidelines in mind, the main one being to convey what had been said as accurately as possible, keeping much of the original flavor. There is no way of separating technique and outcome from the unique personality of each therapist as well as the unique situations existing at the moment. The editor, therefore, used a blue pencil with a fine point. Some incomplete sentences are still incomplete. The pace and style of each therapist come through—all the better for the reader to develop independent conclusions about the relationship between personality and

therapeutic approach, as well as between language and behavior. The editing did attempt to clarify sequence and other practical matters that, left unattended, would make it difficult for the reader to follow the action. Redundancies were reduced, although some were left in because they seemed expressive either of what had taken place or the therapist's state of mind. Many of the questions raised by the listener were included. Some questions and answers were deleted if one or both of the participants meandered from the topic, or if there were forays into interpretation (usually by the listener) that more appropriately belonged in the commentary section.

5. One session was handled differently. An early case, which was thought to have considerable value as a staff learning experience, was presented at a staff conference. The procedure was much the same as with the usual reporting sessions, except that the number of listeners and commentators had been multiplied by a factor of sixteen. In this case (clearly identified in the chapter), the more relevant questions have been preserved, though they come from a variety of colleagues rather than the listener alone.

6. Case selection was also based on obvious criteria. We wanted a good variety of cases, which meant including both men and women (the latter are in about a two-to-one majority at CH as in many other facilities for the aged), people with and without histories of psychiatric problems, long-term and new admissions, the intellectually intact and cognitively disabled, and those representing a wide range of health problems. Included here are several cases that we regard as landmarks in our own work, but others just as rich have been omitted for lack of space. At the time of this writing, the present sampling of cases represents about 15 percent of those seen by the therapist team.

The listener would like to take this opportunity to express his public appreciation for the candor and patience the therapists brought to the reporting sessions. He will long remember these sessions, many of which were intense experiences for both parties. And he will continue to count his blessings for the fact that never, under the greatest provocation, did any of the therapists hurl the tape recorder through the window or haul off and slug the listener. They would have been entitled!

4 REPRESENTATIVE CASES

CASE 1: GINGER S.[1]

by Beverly Ryder

This woman has lived her entire life, since birth, in Massachusetts. She ended her formal education with the eighth grade, later married, and bore two daughters. Ginger's husband died when she was fifty years old; she then lived with one of her daughters until reportedly becoming paranoid after the death of her cat. She was admitted to a state mental hospital and, fifteen years later, came to Cushing. At time of admission, her status was summarized as follows:

1. Bed patient at all times.
2. Deaf, blind, and unable to communicate.
3. Long history of depressive disease with organic brain syndrome.
4. Several decubiti (bed sore).
5. Urinary tract infection (has a catheter).
6. Arteriosclerotic heart disease.
7. Gross tremors of upper extremities.

---

1. Ginger S. was one of the first patients seen in the holistic therapy program. The case was discussed with the listener and then presented at a staff conference; some of the questions and comments from this presentation are included here.

As the record indicates, Ginger S. had been institutionalized for fifteen years and was diagnosed as being totally blind and deaf. According to the staff report, she was unable to communicate except at night when she would cry out in terror. This would sometimes wake up other patients. When anyone would approach her, Ginger would tremble in fear. I was asked to work with her to overcome this fearfulness and help her feel relaxed.

I was also asked to work on her decubitus ulcer. She had a large decubitus ulcer on her right hip and another on her back. Most of the time I concentrated on the right hip.

When I first started working with Ginger, I intuitively felt that she could hear something and could also see somewhat, perhaps faint shadows, but something. I noticed that her area of the ward was dark. One of the first things I did was to pull the shade up so that there would be more light around her. I approached Ginger very gently and touched her on the shoulder and patted her, held her hand.

After I had been working with Ginger for a couple of weeks, she stopped trembling when approached. She remained serene and relaxed. She never spoke, but she communicated in different ways: by expression, by touch, by smiling. She did smile!

I'd touch her hand and she'd give back a feeble little grasp. One day I was talking with her, telling her very candidly how much I cared for her—and with great effort Ginger moved her head and kissed me on the cheek. I can't tell you how overwhelmed I was with that.

Sometimes I would speak to her philosophically, not imposing my philosophy on her but sharing it. I think she enjoyed that. I would sometimes speak about beautiful imaginings. As I was leaving her, I would characteristically tap her on her chin and say, "I wish you beautiful imaginings." I often spoke about imagination to her. One time when I was doing this, she patted my hand. The only thing I can remember is that it was so feeble yet so powerful.

I had a feeling that she had an aphasia problem. I really felt that she could understand but couldn't express that. I believe she understood what I said.

I also felt Ginger would respond to music, but I wasn't sure what kind she'd like. I told her about it beforehand, that I was going to bring her music as a gift. I felt driven to do this. I was going to do it on Sunday, but I felt driven to do it on a Saturday. Friday night I wrote a note to myself, "You must bring music to her tomorrow." And on that tomorrow, that Saturday, one of the birds died—one of my birds that was singing all the time. Her family said she loved animals and became paranoid after her cat died. I told Ginger how I loved my birds and my animals, and I told her I was going to play some music and let my birds sing in the background.

When did her cat die?

Many years ago, when she was first admitted to an institution.

Under what circumstances did the cat die?

I don't know, but there may have been some justification for her paranoid feelings about the cat's death. Someone could have put her cat "to sleep" when Ginger entered the hospital. It happens.

Her history has many gaps in it. There was this bit of information about the cat, and then nothing about her state of mind until she was in a hospital, totally blind and totally deaf, and telling people that she didn't think she belonged there. This was years ago. Her history is very scanty. The blindness and deafness show up as though out of nowhere, perhaps very suddenly. She might have had a cerebrovascular accident (CVA), but this would be guessing. I imagine that it was one of those cases where her daughter couldn't care for her, and a lot of guilt was involved there.

Ginger taught me a lot, and I let her know this. I let her know that she was giving to me as I was giving to her.

I think that it was in May that Ginger had a myocardial infarction. She wasn't expected to survive, but she did. I worked with her late into the evening, stayed with her, helping her to be relaxed, teaching her the purpose of the oxygen, and so forth. Lisa came in at this point also. Ginger would be the first patient that we worked on together, and we worked together right into the evening, particularly when she had trouble breathing.

Were you working at the same or different times?

Most of the time I worked with her. Lisa, maybe you could say something about it.

Lisa: Bev had been there all day and late into the evening. She worked the most with Ginger, and then I stayed with her, and after Bev left I stayed longer. Sometimes it was both of us, sometimes it was one or the other, changing off. Bev and I share a lot of the same experiences—psychic experiences—at the same time, which we thought was unusual.

Shared what kind of experiences?

Lisa: In the middle of the crisis I had my eyes closed, and I saw a man and a woman above Ginger. I said something to Beverly, and she immediately replied, "It's her parents," and I broke out in a cold sweat. I looked over at Bev and she was sweaty, too. It was like everything happened at once. I really felt that Ginger was not in her body at that point. It was strange. I mentioned something to Bev, and she was really surprised because that was what she felt, too.

We also felt around the top of her head. We both felt at the same time a kind of—not a breeze, exactly, but some kind of a force. It felt like a magnetic force. I can't quite explain it. Remember that, Lisa?

Lisa: Every few seconds, really, that rapidly, I'd say something to Bev or she'd say something to me and we'd be just at the right moment. We'd be experiencing the same thing. And we got to laughing about it. We were telling Ginger that we were working together so well, and it was a beautiful experience.

Later, at another time, Ginger had pneumonia with chest congestion and Lisa helped me several times.

This may have been the first time you were working together on a case, but the connection came so easy.

Lisa: There was no if, and, or but.

No effort.

Lisa: It was just amazing.

You hadn't done that before?

Lisa: No, I didn't really know how Bev worked, and she didn't know how I worked. It was really nice. We just accepted what was happening and didn't think to mention it (the shared psychic experience) to anyone.

And Ginger pulled through. However, this episode did undermine her health. There was a slow decline, except that her decubitus ulcer continued to improve. It had started to improve after I worked with her a few weeks. Soon after this, I sensed that Ginger was in pain. I asked her if she hurt. She made a face. So I gently placed my hand on her abdomen and said, "Does it hurt *here*?" This was intuitive on my part, but she nodded yes. I could count on the fingers of one hand the number of times she ever nodded to me. This was an unusual response. All the time that I worked with Ginger I talked right into her ear. I told her I wanted to help her alleviate the pain. I told her a little more about myself, where I was coming from as far as being a healer is concerned. She responded by relaxing. I told Ginger to think back to when she was a young girl, and did some guided images with her. She responded and appeared to be very comfortable and serene. I did tell her that I thought she had a blockage there (beneath the touched place on the abdomen). It was a week later that I was told that Ginger was filled with cancer. I was also told that we couldn't expect her to live longer than two or three months. I stayed with her. I saw her every day. In some ways, her health improved. More and more, our visits were a combination of gentle touch, comforting words, and a sharing of philosophical thoughts and ideas. I consistently left her with the parting words, "I wish you beautiful imaginings." I told her often that I loved her very much, and at such times she would respond with a pat on my hand or a little squeeze. I would tell her although I was going away, say, for the weekend, I was leaving my spirit with her and would take hers with me.

One of the first times I noticed Ginger smiling was on her ninetieth birthday. I felt that she was sometimes chilly around her shoulders, so for her birthday I got her this soft, beautiful, blue blanket and also a card with raised flowers on it. I scented the flowers. This made the card something she could feel and smell. I traced her fingers around the card and read it to her, and let her smell the scent. I gave her flowers, too, and she smelled the flowers and smelled the card. I opened the gift and explained to her that this was to keep her warm and to keep my love around her. I wrapped the blanket around her and kind of tucked her in. I said, "There now, snug as a bug in a rug"—and that was the first time I noticed the smile.

I wonder what effect the blanket had on her night terrors.

Long before that, I had been saying to Ginger that my spirit was with her, that she was not alone. I would say these things close to her ear, and in the same tone I'd say, "It's all right." The blanket added to it, I think, but the process had started much earlier.

In your little philosophical talks with Ginger, was there any way that you insinuated to her that she was dying?

Not until the end. But I did speak to her about another dimension that developed between us. I found that I would dream of Ginger, like I do with a lot of my patients. Once I told her about the dream I had about her. During this dream she appeared to me healthy, standing up, beautiful. It was a beautiful dream and I told her, and this elicited an emotional response from her. Her eyes filled up, and she patted my hand, which I think was absolutely all her body could let her do.

I want to ask about the night screaming. Is there any connection about your dreaming about Ginger and her sleeping well without the screaming?

She stopped screaming almost within the second week I worked with her.

Had you started dreaming about her then, in those first two weeks?

Yes, I did.

I was wondering if there was a time correlation there.

It could be.

I'll tell you the feeling I got when she smiled, and her eyes kind of teared up. My feeling was that she was trying to get through to me in that way. When I was telling her about the dream, the way she responded—a feeling came over me. I felt she did this deliberately, I mean, on purpose, a message, that she somehow *provoked* the dream. It was as if she were telling me she was all right. I had this feeling somewhat from the dream itself, and this was reinforced by the way she reacted when I told her of the dream.

Her condition, especially in her lungs, gradually became worse. The lungs filled. She had to be suctioned. For a while her kidneys backed up and she had severe edema. So I'd be concentrating from one area to the other. I went from concentrating on her lungs to her kidneys and so forth. During that time, whatever area I was concentrating on improved after I had been with her. Her kidneys got better, but then something else got worse. I would place my hand on her chest because she had difficulty breathing with her lungs filled.

Even the congestion would somehow subside. I always explained to Ginger that *her* thought helped, her thinking with me helped. It was her response to what I was doing that had the healing effect. I really believe she understood; she always understood.

Near the end of the time when I would visit her, toward the end, just before she died, Ginger slept a lot more. But even while she was sleeping, there was a response. That's sort of hard to define. I just could *feel* her respond. I always, always felt welcome. Ginger was always serene, calm, relaxed, accepting. In fact, I spent more time with her than I had before, sharing more and more of my love with her, my thoughts on life and so forth. I spoke of God, love. I spoke of us being one with the universe, yet alone in our ways of perceiving things. I felt she welcomed this, that this is what she wanted to hear and think about.

There was then a long weekend because of the Columbus Day holiday. It was also my daughter's birthday, and I had planned on some activities at home. I went into the hospital Sunday so I could be with Ginger for a couple of hours. When I arrived there, she looked amazingly healthy. The color was back. She looked peaceful and calm. I noticed she didn't have the oxygen. This was easy to notice because lately she had had it constantly. I stayed with her for a while. When I talked with her she was responsive and squeezed my hand when I spoke my thoughts about suffering and how I hoped that her suffering would be over. I told Ginger how much I loved her and cared for her, that I would always be there for her. I told her that my soul and my spirit would always welcome her—and that if that was something she didn't want, that was all right, too. I told her again the date and time. I told her I was there on Sunday because I wouldn't be in the next day; it was my daughter's birthday. Oh, by the way, she had met my daughter. Barbie sometimes would visit with her on weekends when I couldn't. She would tell Ginger who she was, and Ginger would pat her hand. That was a ritual.

As I was talking with her, Ginger began to have a difficult time breathing. I got even closer to her, almost held her, told her it's all right, I'm here. For maybe fifteen minutes, maybe half an hour, it was as if time were suspended. There was nothing but myself and Ginger. Nothing existed but ourselves. And I believe in it as something divine with us, a kind of sharing. I just talked as the words came to me, intuitively, continually, words of encouragement, saying to her, "It's all right, it's all right." And I felt an enormous strength go through me to her. And then something even more interesting happened. *I felt a strength going from her to me, at the same time.* I really felt at one with her. I believe we were, in a sense, one. I felt myself taking her or her essence, whatever it is, spiritually, lifting her, giving her strength. And yet it was very strange: at the same time, she was giving me strength.

I didn't dare leave her for a moment, because I felt that each breath that she took might be her last one. I was also telling her to relax: "It's all right, it's all right." I was saying things like, "If I have ever offended you, please forgive me because I don't know—sometimes I might have offended you without meaning to." That was the only time that Ginger seemed a little disturbed, and she gave me another squeeze. I said to her, "I think you need some oxygen. I'm going to get the nurse, to get you some oxygen." All this time, Ginger had her eyes closed. After I said this to Ginger, she seemed to calm down, relax, and her breathing was just slightly better. As I was coming back from the getting the nurse, something happened that I felt was rather extraordinary. Ginger still had her eyes closed but she lifted her hand up for me to take. That was the most extraordinary thing! It was just as I was coming close to her—she just lifted her hand right up for me to take. She had never done that before. When I took Ginger's hand she had more strength than ever. When she held my hand—the squeeze she gave me, the returning—it was more than ever.

That was amazing. It was totally unexpected, totally. I was taken aback. It almost disoriented me for a few minutes when I felt that strength. I didn't know where it was coming from and then I just went with it, with the strength that I felt coming from her, whatever it was. I held her, kissed her on the forehead, and told her, "I love you so." I told her this over and over again. The nurse was there and was trying to adjust the oxygen. Ginger, however, breathed with her mouth opened. She consistently did this. I asked the nurse if the oxygen was going to help Ginger with her mouth open. At this moment it seemed crucial that she have the oxygen. The nurse said she didn't think it would help much if Ginger kept her mouth open. I said, "Well, I'll encourage her to close her mouth; I'll do the best I can." The nurse kind of laughed a little because a lot of people still did not believe that Ginger could hear.

I talked right into her ear. I apologized for making this demand on her because I knew how weak she was. I said, "Ginger, you must close your mouth and breath through your nose to get the benefit of this oxygen. You need the oxygen. It's going to help you breathe better. Breathe through your nose, Ginger." At first there was no response. I still stayed with her. I must have repeated these suggestions for two or three minutes. And then she did—she closed her mouth, closed it rather tightly, sniffed a couple of times, then started breathing through her nose. I was really pleased to see this response, and the nurse was quite startled. I mean, *startled*. I thought the nurse was going to faint. She actually turned pale, the nurse did, right before my eyes. The nurse said, "I don't believe that," because it was very evident that Ginger was responding to the suggestion.

She couldn't maintain it, though. She just didn't have the strength to keep her life going. I said to Ginger, "It's all right, it's all right. I know you don't have much strength." I patter her gently and stayed with her for about another hour. When I left, I told her that I would see her on Tuesday. I told Ginger that I loved her dearly and that my spirit would always be open to her. She died twelve hours later.

I was sleeping and the phone rang, and they told me that Ginger had died. I was glad I was at home—away—for selfish reasons, I guess, because I just couldn't control myself. As soon as I hung up, I wept, wept, and wept. For hours. I wept for the years she was institutionalized, the years she had no one to relate to. I wept for her family, for all that they had missed, because she gave something that was beautiful, just beautiful. I wept, too, because I'm going to miss her for a long time. I guess I don't know all the reasons. I still find myself thinking of Ginger when I drive home, and I still weep, just a little bit. I guess that's just how it's going to be.

Lisa: The nurses believed Ginger was going to die four or five different times, and they would keep telling this to her.

I'm glad you brought this up. I was with Ginger a few days before she did pass away, and I'd be getting these looks from some nurses. It was almost an accusing look, as if I were keeping her alive beyond the call of humanism. In my mind, this was not what I was doing. I was trying to help Ginger feel comfortable. There was one particular time when I was requesting something for her; I was asking if she could be suctioned. She needed it. "Well," a nurse said, "we just suctioned her, and it will just have to be done again!" That was her response. I was standing on this side of Ginger and the nurse was on the other side of her. I said, "Well, if it's not too much trouble, it might relieve her so her breathing will be more comfortable." The nurse said, "Well, what Ginger needs is to go home," meaning death. I just looked at the nurse and patted Ginger on the shoulder, trying to make a mental communication with her. Then I said something like, "I plan on being with her on the weekend. I'll probably come in on Sunday because I came in on last Sunday." The nurse said, "Let's hope she isn't here by Sunday." I managed to control myself. At that point I felt angry, but I said nothing. The nurse left and I bent close to Ginger's ear and said, "You can live as long as you want to live. I'm right here." She had a smile on her face. I'll never forget it. It was like a secret being shared.

When Ginger died, the nurses said she had peace, that her face was very peaceful and calm.

There are a few things I didn't mention. I would try to help Ginger eat by having her pretend she was at a picnic when she was a little girl. She seemed to understand this, and her eating did become easier. This was before her final decline. I don't know whether I should add this or not, but a couple of the nurses who worked with her throughout the whole time would tell her I was coming when Ginger was in discomfort, and they told me she responded to that. "Bev will be here later" or "Bev will be here tomorrow." They would say this when they had to bathe or move her, and this might have caused Ginger some pain; and they wouldn't have said this if they didn't think it did some good.

What would you do when she was sleeping?

I would stand by her, just look at her, and think about how much I cared about her.

Would you touch her?

Sometimes I would. Just gently lay my hand on her shoulder so it wouldn't wake her up, touch her shoulder and once in a while pat her.

I have been making notes on all the ways she responded to you, and I would like to go over them. There was the blanket and touch, the card and touch, plus the fragrance of the card, and—

And the rose.

Two senses involved there. The tap on the hand became the squeeze of the hand. There was the nod of her head, also the smile, and her lifting her hand at the end. Now is there anything else I missed?

Once she did say one word. She said "yes" once. I felt she was thirsty. It was intuitive. I said, "Would you like a drink of water?" There was no response. I saw beside her what I thought was orange juice and I said, "How would you like some orange juice, some nice, fresh orange juice?" She said "yes" then. Yes was the only word she ever said. By the way, it turned out to be grapefruit juice, and she didn't like it.

I was wondering about the situation when you were trying to persuade her to breathe through her nose so the oxygen would be effective. You repeated your request for two or three minutes. Was she having trouble in registering what you were saying?

She didn't have the strength. That was the main thing.

Suppose that a person like Ginger has not had the practice of responding to people for a long time, over a period of years. As a result she has to rebuild this ability. When she finds someone close to her, or someone gets close to her, this rapport might be what she needs to overcome all the accumulated inhibitions and resistance to talking.

She did try to talk. She would make attempts every once in a while. And she would also perk her ear. You could see that. She was very interested in the time and data and things like what was happening around her, and she would also perk her ear when I talked philosophically.

If she didn't like the philosophy, I think you would have picked it up. She would have given some sign.

Socked me or something.

Did you look into her background to see what interests she had?

Yes, but I couldn't find anything. That's what I felt was so pitiful. But that she heard me, there is no doubt.

Andrea: She had heard the nurses at night talking about her death. She was so scared that she would cry out at night.

The whole time I was with her, the whole eight months, she didn't cry out. Another thing: they said she would live only two or three months. The doctor said, "Don't even think of three months because that would be extraordinary." That was in May, and she died October 8. I think I gave her the option of deciding when her death would be.

The nurses became attached to her, too. I feel that it spilled over, there was a kind of spillover effect. The nurses could see me talking to her, treating her like an intelligent person who could understand. First there were looks like I was out of my nut, and then things started happening. I would go in, for example, and go from one side of the bed to the other and she would turn her head and the nurse would say, "She's looking at you! She's hearing you!" This was at the beginning.

A couple of times she cuddled, that's another thing. When I would hold her hand, her whole self would sort of cuddle to my hand. She didn't do that all the time, but every once in a while.

I think that *everybody* has an immeasurable amount of love to give. So many feel it's not the right thing to do. If we could let them know it! Let them know that certainly it *is* the right thing to do. If other people can recognize how real and how important and how right loving is, that will make the difference.

Lisa: When somebody says, "It's okay, it's okay," that makes the difference. Many people can love but they just seem to need the permission.

CASE 2: DORIS G.

by Lisa B. Hathaway

Doris G. was born in a small town in Massachusetts. Her only sibling, a sister, died in infancy, and her mother died when Doris was twelve years old. After graduating from a business college, she worked as a bookkeeper until suffering a heart attack in her sixty-eighth year. She remained in a rest home for two or three months and then went back to work.

She continued to live in her own home for another dozen years. Doris G. had never married and had no known relatives, but she had many friends throughout the years. She was described as a bright and knowledgeable woman with interests in national and world politics.

Following years of reasonably good health, she developed leg ulcers and was admitted to a local hospital. She was noted to be somewhat confused at this time. After discharge she returned to her home despite suffering "dizzy spells." She managed for more than another year until she fell at home and fractured her left hip. This time after her treatment at a local hospital, she was admitted directly to Cushing Hospital.

When she entered Cushing Hospital at eighty-two years of age, Doris G. was found to have degenerative arthritis in both knees, central macular degeneration, intermittent atrial arrhythmia (by history), chronic brain syndrome, and multiple seizures with probable cerebrovascular accident (CVA). These were in addition to the recent hip fracture from which she had not completely recovered.

I started working with Doris G. soon after she arrived at Cushing. She had a great deal of pain associated with the hip fracture and the degenerative arthritis in her knees. I was working with her for that reason. I wanted to relieve the pain and comfort her as much as possible.

What I want to tell you about is a specific incident. She had fourteen seizures in a matter of a few hours. The first seizure came after lunch. She complained then of blurred vision. A little later she had another seizure. I was called at my home. The operator said, "There is a patient dying on Ward D." The operator didn't say a name. I never would have thought that it was Doris. As I arrived, they were wheeling her to the Intensive Care Unit, and we all arrived at the same time. The nurses did what they had to do as far as getting her comfortable and settling her in as a new admission on that ward. The priest popped in for barely twenty seconds and did his routine, said a little prayer.

What did he actually do?

He did the sign of the cross and said a few words—like, two sentences—and went out the other door. I couldn't believe it. It wasn't like, "Hi, Doris." It wasn't like he knew her or wanted to know her. It was just like this was his duty. He came in, gave a certain prayer, and left. I was so shocked because I thought for sure he'd be in there for a long time.

Did he address her by name?

Yes, he did say, "Doris G." He said her name, and said just a few words more, and then he was gone. It was so short I just couldn't believe what I was seeing.[2]

How did Doris G. respond to what was going on at this time?

Just staring. Everything was happening much too fast, and not a heck of a lot was being explained to her. "This woman has had two grand mal seizures already!" Everybody was going every which way, trying to figure out the best thing to do, and nobody was with Doris. They were all running in and out.

So I went in there and stayed with her for about two and a half hours. During this time she had the other twelve seizures—grand mal seizures, one after the other. Within the first forty minutes she was in most of them almost continuously. She'd just get out of one and she'd slide into another. It was really intense.

I asked her if she had any pain. She looked at me and said, "No." Then she realized that out of all the people in her room at that time there was someone she knew, which was me, and she looked relieved. I stayed with her throught the seizures, one after another, until she reached fourteen. During the whole time I held her head lovingly with both hands for protection. I spoke to her often, using soft, soothing words, suggesting good things and suggesting relaxation. I threw everything I could possibly think of into helping this woman.

---

2. This chaplain has since been replaced.

Immediately I felt I had to protect her head. I felt protection was very important. While she was going through these intense seizures—her whole body was going through them—I'd talk to her very calmly. I spoke to her about what was happening. "It's all right, Doris. Relax your body. Relax your body from your head to your toes." I'd speak very softly and say the same thing over and over. "This is almost over, Doris. It's okay. It will never be like this again. The worst will soon be over."

Had you ever used this procedure with her for other purposes?

No, this was the first time.

So this means that you tried to teach her relaxation procedures and use imagery—for the first time—while she was in the middle of a whole series of seizures. The odds seemed to be stacked against success for both reasons—the seizures and the fact you had not tried them with her before.

I did have something going for me. I was trying to heal her knees, and she wanted this very much. When she came into Cushing she said, "This is only temporary. I'm going back to my home as soon as my hip and knees heal." I had just been working with her a couple of weeks before the seizures came.

On that day I stayed with her about seven hours. After I had been with her for about two and a half hours, I kept popping in and out. I'd constantly tell her where she was, what was happening to her body, and that she'd be fine, she'd recover completely. If she didn't feel right, I told her it was because of the medication: "It will wear off, and you will be fine." At 9:10 p.m. the ward called me. They said that she was responding to people but in a kind of grunting moan. It was really scary. They asked me to come down because they figured a familiar face would be really helpful at this point. When I reached Doris I felt that her condition was becoming much more stable. She woke up groaning and scared frequently. I had one hand on hers and the other on her forehead, saying, "It's all right, Doris; it's okay. You're still at Cushing Hospital but in a different room." I said it over and over again. She'd keep waking up and forget what I had said before, but I knew the repetition was important. She'd always be relieved after I said it, then drift off for a moment, then wake up again. I said, "You've had some seizures that you've never experienced before, but you're okay now. The medication makes you feel funny, but it's okay. It will pass. The medication will wear off. You're not alone." Each time she recognized me with a little more clarity. She listened to me as I spoke. After about an hour and twenty minutes she squeezed my hand as I spoke to her.

I knew that she was scared, but what really bothered me was that she couldn't form words yet, was unable to communicate—and that must have been scaring her, too. "What's this sound coming out of my mouth?" She must have been thinking, wondering if it was going to be permanent. The doctor was aware of her apprehension. I left at about one o'clock in the morning, but the doctor still didn't want to give her a sedative because they didn't know the extent of any damage that the seizures might have done. Her vital signs had been stable for eight hours, but she had not slept at all and continued to attempt to communicate only by a startled kind of sound.

The next day, Doris could respond to the nurses by blinking and squeezing her hand, but she was as yet nonverbal. I could see the torment in her eyes. She wanted so badly to speak, to form words. The nurse asked if I could get a response as to whether or not she had pain. I said, "Doris, do you have any pain?" And to the amazement of all, she said, just as loud and clear, "I don't know." The tears came to my eyes as they came to her eyes. I could literally feel the torment that was within her, and sympathize with her.

You felt so strongly for Doris. If you could put her feelings into words, what do you think she would say at that time?

Just totally helpless, totally vulnerable, absolutely no control, no strength whatsoever—just, "I'm here. What has happened? What will happen next?" And it was just that look in her eyes, that burning, full of tears, a really devastated kind of feeling. As though a bomb had just gone off, something totally unexpected. I could feel the loss within her.

I explained again what had happened to her, and I told her, "You'll be able to speak. Have patience with yourself, have patience. You've been through a lot." I constantly tried to express what I thought she was thinking at the time, what was bothering her. I said, "You know, Doris, it's harder to receive than it is to give: I believe that. And I believe that you're a giver and a doer—there's nothing wrong with that. It's just your turn now to receive. I care about you so very much. I'm sending you a lot of loving thoughts along with a healing." Then she wriggled out a smile. You can tell she wanted to cry, just as a sign of relief.

I told her that her speech was going to become easier each time, her memory clearer and sharper. "You have to be patient with yourself, Doris, there's plenty of time. I know that you would like to speak to me. I know that you can hear me. Don't worry."

I explained to her about the catheter that they were going to insert in her. That way she wouldn't have to fuss with the embarrassment of bed pans. She hates bed pans and commodes and anything to do with that, so she refused to drink because that would make her go. She has a lot of embarrassment with that. She has a fear of being incontinent. I asked Doris to promise me she would try and sleep. She shook her head and said, "Yes."

The nurses' notes the next morning said that she appeared more alert, speaking in short phrases, moving arms, having a good swallow reflex, but very anxious, appearing frightened upon approach; more relaxed in p.m., skin warm and dry, no seizures or symptoms of seizure activity noted. She had difficulty expressing her needs and became frustrated and anxious easily.

It took about three days for Doris to get fully back to sentences again. At first it was a word or two, then it got to be four-word sentences and then—bang!—it came back on the third day. She was concerned then about her memory: "I can't remember." I told her that she would remember; the condition was only temporary. I said, "Don't fight it; it's going to come back before you know it. You've just got to let it come when your body is ready to give it back to you." I told her how beautiful she was. Before, she could never accept that. She'd say, "Now, that's silly! I'm not beautiful; don't you tell me things like that!" But at this point I felt that she would accept it.

The supervisory nurse came in and told me that it was an absolute miracle that Doris had come back so far at this point. But the real intense work came afterward, bringing her back to reality, helping her memory. She had pain. After the healing, she said the pain was gone, and she was moving her arms and sitting up. She was really progressing, but lots of problems arose. She's alert and clear in her speech, but her memory gives her problems. Doris said once, "Has my father been here? Is he still alive? I saw him at the door, but I couldn't get out of bed to see him. No—of course, he is dead. All of my family is dead. I'm single, of course, no children."

I explained that the image of her father was real—as an image. Many people see apparitions. It does not mean that she has lost her mind. She seemed surprised but then relieved. She has partial memory for her seizure episode. "I remember the pain, and then I couldn't eat, and then I had the seizures. They said I had visitors, but I don't remember." "That's not your fault," I told her, "You were under medication to control your seizures, and at the same time this made things hazy." I asked if she had any pain in her legs now. No, she didn't. Does she remember when I used to work with her to relieve the pain and swelling? Yes, she does.

Dr. Z. said that she was progressing beautifully, but not to be surprised if she does die because her heart is bad.

Doris is the Last Leaf of the Tree. I just remembered that! She shared a dream with me. "I had a dream that you asked me to draw what I remembered. But I don't know what happened to the drawing." That's what she said. The funny thing is that she doesn't know that I have any association with art whatsoever. She knew me but not my name. She doesn't know that I'm an expressive therapist and a person who does art.

She also told me how she "died for a while." I told her it was natural for a person who had gone through what she did to have that kind of experience: "Don't be frightened by it." I kept telling her specifically that, yes, she will remember, her memory will return just as well as her speech has. Beverly and I reinforced the positive with her constantly. Bev was telling Doris the exact same things I was—word for word—and yet we never discussed this beforehand. We just naturally seem to do the same things.

Doris felt it was important to explain to me that she received Sheila as her Christian name, but her mother's name was Doris.

Perhaps by taking her mother's name this gave her a kind of continuity within the family, since she is the Last Leaf. . . . As she was describing her experiences during the seizures—what she remembers of it—did she mention anything of what's now considered the classic after-life experience: dark tunnels, radiant beings of light, and that sort of thing?

No. She was just trying to put the experience together, one sentence at a time. "I died, you know. I remember my father at the door." She wouldn't get any more words out for a minute or two, and every once in a while—bang!—a sentence would come out. Finally she said, "Well, my father's been dead a long time." She'd just go back and forth in her thoughts, and I'd just let her talk; I didn't want to interrupt that flow that she was in.

She was more interested in talking with you about the experience and getting her thoughts together than in conveying a cohesive story?

Right. Exactly. She was confused at that point—fleeting moments of knowing what was what.

I want to share some of the things she said to me during the next couple of weeks. She said, "Boy, do I dream a lot!" I told her how terrific it is for her to dream. "Last night was the first night that I slept till morning." She said that and felt really good about it. She told us that she loves it when Beverly and I visit. "When you get old, your friends seem to disappear. Thanks *so much* for taking the time to come and see me."

These days she is very concerned about her house. A family that is very close to her is taking care of it for her. She is worried about the pipes freezing and that sort of thing.

These are realistic concerns.

Yes, 100 percent. Who is going to pay the bills? Who is going to clean? Who is going to make sure the windows are locked up for the winter? She is back to reality with all of the everyday problems. By the way, she even called Dr. Z. by his right name this morning. He used to ask her every day; it was sort of a game between them. Now she has it right and is very proud of it. She does get Beverly and me confused at times because we do very much the same things. I explained to her that the staff and patients will begin to look familiar to her. "That part of your brain that recalls things is healing very well. Have patience; you will remember." I also reminded her that her original goal is to be rehabilitated to walk. Oh, now she remembers my name, and Bev's name, as well as Dr. Z.'s.

How far away are we in time from the seizures?

Fifteen days. She does not have her glasses at this point. I know that she used to love to write, being a bookkeeper. She has tiny little printing, and I encourage her to write the names of people she knows. She is also doing the alphabet and numbers. Her glasses were broken, I think, and she doesn't have a replacement yet. This makes it difficult for her to use writing as a tool to improve her memory.

There has been another problem. Her left knee has doubled in size compared with the photographs I had taken earlier. She no longer has trouble with her right leg. I felt that it wasn't the arthritis, but a whole different thing inside of her knee. I didn't know what throm-bitis was, though. At this point, the head nurse said that there was a possibility of her having thrombitis, so Heparin was ordered to thin the blood, and she was given some other medication for this, too. Now the thrombitis is controlled by medication, and she doesn't have any more problems with her knees. Her long-term memory is back, but she has trouble hanging onto events in short-term memory.

I stopped working with her because the problems I was there to help her with are under control. I still see her a lot, and Bev sees her. We reinforce the good things she does. She is just an incredible lady. She went through a heck of a lot.

CASE 3: JOHN Z.

by Beverly Ryder

This seventy-six-year-old man, married and with one son, was admitted to Cushing Hospital directly from his home. Athletic when younger, he particularly enjoyed swimming. He was employed as a truck driver throughout much of his life and worked on cars as a hobby. He was active in a golden age club after his retirement and did a lot of travelling with this group.

Six diagnoses were made upon his admission: chronic brain syndrome; carcinoma of prostate (history); transitional cell carcinoma, bladder; brain stem stroke cerebrovascular accident (CVA) (history); gangrene of both feet (present), and pneumonia (present). He was admitted directly to the Intensive Care Unit (ICU) because of the pneumonia and gangrene.

The first time I began working with John was a time when I was on the ICU to see another patient. The nurse came over and asked if I'd be willing to work with a new patient who had a very severe problem of gangrene in both feet. There was a possibility that his feet might have to be amputated. He had already had surgery at another hospital to try to improve circulation in one of his legs. I'm not sure exactly what that was all about. I said, "Sure, I would be glad to."

He was in the solarium, sitting on one of those long chairs that you can wheel, a lounging-type chair. He looked rather peaceful. His eyes—there's something that happens in that first meeting when I look directly into the person's eyes and something transpires that I just can't define very well, but it's something very special. That very special thing happened with him, sort of an *understanding*. This can happen no matter what the degree of brain damage, and it happened this time. I wasn't aware of how much brain damage he had at that time.

"Hello!" I introduced myself to him. He said hello to me. And then I was struck with the odor! The gangrene odor! I looked at his feet. I'd worked in nursing homes and I had never seen anything quite like that, not that bad. His feet were really bad. There were many wide areas of black, and there was stuff oozing out. A part of me said, "Oh, God, what can be done?" And another part of me became transformed. I just relaxed and felt confident that something could be done.

I was still divided within myself, though. One part of me was very positive, but another part of me was different. I had a conflict when I looked at his feet. If I was going to be logical, then I had to wonder if anything could be done.

At this moment there wasn't just one nurse there; several had gathered and they were all looking at me, anticipating how I would react. They had that holding-their-breaths sort of look: Is she going to be able to handle this? It presented me with a challenge.

I looked at John and said, "John, I think I can help you, help you so your feet will heal. But you'll have to work with me. We'll work together." I also said that I was something of a healer. I wasn't too happy with myself that I had said this. I quickly modified it. I told him that if he were willing to work with me that I felt that he would get better. I would ask him to imagine some things and to think along with me. He just nodded, and I thought he understood—and I still think he did, to this day. Now, mind you, I did not know the severity of his brain damage; I had just met him.

I also told John that I was going to keep him in my heart. He was going to be in my prayers. I wasn't going to touch the areas that were afflicted. My hand would be above the areas sometimes, though, and I was going to do that because I wanted him to think along with me. I wanted his blood to flow down to the sick area. He was going to bring fresh blood in there and keep building it up, helping the area to heal. He nodded. Yep, he really did.

And so, at that first meeting, I did what might traditionally be called a healing. My hands passed over his legs—from the knees down to the feet, and concentrating around the feet. The idea of my hand going from the knee down to the feet was for circulation. At the same time I imagined a healing process going on. I imagined his feet as new feet. I told John I wanted him to imagine this, too. I'd like him to picture in his mind his feet as they were when he was a young man.

As I was doing this, the nurses came around. They stood around me and they—very shyly—held each other's hands in a circle around me. They bowed their heads. I did the same. I would occasionally look at John's eyes. I was sort of going in and out of a trance-like state.

I was working with him approximately fifteen minutes a day; about five minutes of this was devoted to healing, the rest was general talking and relating. The nurses stood there like that, and each one of the nurses sort of meditated or prayed silently in her own way. I heard a couple of "Please, dear God" sort of things, a whispering. This must have made a profound impression on him. It made a profound impression on me. Once when I was standing there meditating and imagining his feet getting better, one of the nurses took my hand and one took the other hand, and they made me part of the circle. This surprised me a little—it did—and I thought it was beautiful. I was still fairly new; the nurses and I really hadn't had much chance to know each other or for them to find out exactly what I was doing. This incident came soon after I had been working with Ginger (Case 1). There was an improvement with her, and so I think they felt a certain confidence in me. Most of the nurses there, on that ward, are into Charismatic Christianity. They believe very much in spiritual healings and absent healings, that sort of thing. It was helpful to my work there that they had this kind of belief.

I asked John—I always do this with the people I see—I asked John if he would like me to come back and he said, "Yes."

Had you given him your name right away?

Yes, I've disciplined myself to do that almost all the time with most of my patients, particularly patients who have problems with memory. "It's me again. It's Beverly. It's Beverly." A couple of times he did say my name. Even to this day, though, I don't think he knows all the time what my name is. However, when he sees me—a big smile! If's he's staring off into space, I walk around him and look into his eyes. As soon as they meet mine there's a smile and he really lights up, a kind of radiated smile. "Oh, it's you, it's you!" he'll say. It's rather phenomenal because he'll do this even if he's in one of his moods where he's being rather irritable. Nursing might be giving him a hard time. If I walk in, he responds in this lighting-up, cheering-up way. He's very consistent. This is true even now, when I don't work with him as closely as I did before.

I'd like to get back to the first visits. After I saw John that day, he did indicate that he wanted me to come back. I told him it would be hard work. "This business of getting well—it's hard work, but we can do it together." I was just beginning to sense the problems he was having with his brain damage. After that, I read his thoughts and became more sensitive to the damage that he had from his CVAs.

His wife's attitude was very interesting. She accepted the fact that his feet were healing and attributed this to nursing and myself. She thought it was miraculous, though she didn't have trouble accepting it. But yet, as far as his state of mind was concerned, she wasn't willing to have even a tiny bit of hope. "No, he doesn't remember me. The doctor says he can't think right." She was very strong about that. I tried to show her, but she would always interpret his behavior as hopeless.

Did she have any investment in wanting him to stay impaired mentally?

I had to draw that conclusion, I had to. She did take care of him for many years, and this was very difficult for her. Perhaps she was afraid that if he got better that way, too—his mind as well as his body—then she'd have to take him back and have that burden again. I was sensitive to the problem that she must have had in anticipating him getting well altogether because it was clear that she wanted him to get well physically. She didn't want to see him amputated, and she was very grateful that this didn't have to happen after all. So I thought a lot about this, why she didn't see this improvement in his ability to relate even when it was clearly there. It was really phenomenal. It (the improvement) would be staring her right in the face. I tried to point it out to her, but that made her upset. She told me that I was misinterpreting. That could be. But as time went by it didn't take any interpreting. John became more coherent; he began to talk in sentences. He would reminisce about his life and show himself really to be there, and his wife continued to treat him very much as if he were a child. She pushed that.

Were you and his wife ever together with John when he was behaving in a more rational way, so that you both were seeing and hearing the same thing, but she was denying it?

Yes. This is when I realized that she must have a real problem and that I would have to respect this and just work the best I could with him anyhow. It was a time when he was reminiscing. I had asked him a question about whether he had ever fixed cars. "Oh, yes, many times. If you ever have a problem, bring your car to me; I'll do what I can." It was this kind of interaction, even a little beyond this. I was trying to ask him questions he could answer. She denied that this had been anything like a conversation; she was adamant about it.

Did she speak about him in the third person when he was right there?

Yes, she did. I run into this all the time with families, and even with nursing. I don't say anything directly to them. I just play-act a little. His wife and some nurses are saying things like: "John is really not doing well. He's not sleeping. He's not eating. He's bothering everybody." I say *to him*: "Is that right, John? Are you feeling bad? It's almost as if I'm being a little rude to the people who are talking *about* him and not *to* him. Rather than speak my mind to them directly, I take these opportunities to speak directly to the patient. I do this even if the person supposedly can't respond. I did this with Ginger who was listed and treated as blind and deaf. Sometimes this is very effective, and sometimes not. And sometimes it makes the other person feel a little uneasy. Sometimes I'll suggest that we talk to the person together: "Let's ask John." Are we treating this man as a person or a nonperson? If he is on the borderline because of dementia, or organic brain syndrome, then the way we treat him might well make the difference.

I think this is a crucial variable. It goes back to that initial eye contact with the individual. You treat the person right from the start as if at least a part of him comprehends what you are doing and what you are saying, although he may not be able to express this. If we didn't do this, I doubt very much that we'd be successful in working with patients. It's almost an unconditional part of what we're doing. We start treating people as people right from the start and never stop. I also respect the problems that go along with brain damage. This is a challenge, and it's something that you have to take into consideration, the cognitive aspect of it. For example, when I was working with John on his circulation, I was careful to explain why I asked him to imagine certain things. Not only would I ask him to imagine the sun beating on his feet, shining on his feet, his feet becoming warmer and warmer, but I would also explain why, and why it would help him. I would do this in the simplest terms possible. For example, I told him about Davey, my son, and how I used these techniques with him. I told him about the armies in his blood that are fighting for his health. "John, when you imagine the sun shining on your feet, there is a good reason why your feet are going to feel warmer. It's because more blood is going to the area, and this blood is bringing strength from the rest of your body, fresh and healing. The blood is helping your body rebuild your skin."

I was also working with him on relaxation. They said he had become very agitated and was bothering other patients. I went in one day and said, "We are going to work on relaxation now. We are going to do some breathing exercises. You will relax and that will make you feel better." I started the relaxation technique. He looked at me and said, "What do you mean, *relax*? I don't know what you mean." I said, "I'm so glad you told me that, John. Whenever you don't understand, please tell me." Then I said, "Let's see now, John, what is to relax? Think back to when you were working. You're driving a truck. You've had a hard day driving." I made sure he was following along with these images. "Do you remember working really hard and coming home from work exhausted?" "Yes, I remember that." "Do you have a favorite chair that you sit in?" "Yes." "Just imagine you are sitting in that chair. Remember how you felt after that hard day's work, finally getting a chance just to sit in your favorite comfortable chair." John became so excited. He said, "Oh, that's it! *That's* what it's like to relax!" He was happy and pleased with himself that he could use his mind in this way. And that was quite a thing, with the brain damage he had.

From that time on, I did not have much difficulty in helping him to relax. There were times when it did take a lot of work; it was a challenge.

His feet begin to heal rather rapidly, faster than they had anticipated. At the time his feet were healing, I was also encouraging him to eat. I explained this in sort of an educational way, how important it was that he had the fresh protein to rebuild his feet. John's appetite improved, his spirit improved, his general well-being. He became less agitated, and his feet healed day by day.

I would like to go back for just a moment. About a week after my initial visit with John I had a dream of him. I dreamed that I saw him completely healed. He doesn't look at all his age; he looks a lot younger. His skin is soft and young-looking. You would not imagine he is the age he is. And in this dream I could see him just walking. John actually did get so well at one point that he did walk. I told him that I had this dream because it was something good to share with him. A little later on I had another dream of him. This is a type of dream I rarely have. I feel that maybe in experiencing the dreams, this would have an effect at the hospital, a positive effect on the healing process.

Did he share any of his dreams with you?

No. But he did start doing something that I thought was interesting. I have not seen him do this with any other individual, and I'm often there when there are other people around. He asked me how *I* am.

John probably was able to respond to the relaxation technique because there was a healing process going on. People sometimes forget that there is healing after a CVA; it is possible to compensate and improve even though damage has been done. That just might be why it happened.

John's legs were documented as completely healed two months after the initial contact, and he was moved to Ward C. At this point, not only were his feet completely healed and his appetite keen but he was much calmer. He was more in control. He would become agitated at times, but it was controllable: you could talk to him about it, and he would calm down. But as soon as he went to Ward C he slipped right back, even with me. He became more disoriented. He had difficulty remembering me for the first two times I went to see him there. The third time, though, he remembered me and came more alive. I told him I would come to see him there also. But there was a time that I didn't see him as often as before. He got sick again and went back to ICU. They called me in on it again. He's been in ICU since, and he's been doing fine.

Will you describe the differences between these two wards during the times John was there?

Actually, it was the first time I was introduced to Ward C myself. I had never been down there. Can I speak candidly? When I entered the ward I was really horrified. I really was. I was horrified because everyone appeared to be so isolated. All the men were lying down in their chairs, very little action. Staffing was minimal.

It's not like that now. It's much better now. That must have been a particularly difficult time.

I am talking about that one side of the ward. It seemed to me, to use a poor expression, that everybody was just vegetating. I was struck with John being so disoriented and not recognizing me. I sat with John and talked with him. Though he responded, I knew he didn't recognize me. He didn't have the old smile and the "It's you!" As I said, it wasn't till the third time that the recognition returned. But he seemed so sad. He seemed so isolated and lonely and sad.

It was really strange. There he was just staring off in space with nothing to do, nothing to interact with. A lot of them were all together like that.

Was the ward unusually crowded?

Yes, it was. Some patients were amusing themselves by making strange noises, and others were doing all kinds of things. It's no wonder. It's just no wonder because if you are sitting and having no one to talk to. . . . I didn't notice the staff interacting with them at all that time. This may have changed since then.

What happened was that the same thing started happening to John's legs again. The skin began to break down; it was in the beginning stage of gangrene. So, physically he has deteriorated very quickly. I think this is what happened from my side of it: I kept seeing him, but not as often because he was supposedly healed. I should have followed my own feelings more and continued to see him often. I received a referral from Dr. Z. of the impending gangrene and went back to working with John.

What is his condition now?

It's very good; however, he's not walking. I feel that we could work toward that goal if there were a lot of time I could devote to him. But now I'm running into problems on priorities. There are other patients at different points in their conditions and in my work with them. There are some others who also need me a lot right now. I don't know how to say this. It's almost like you have to put a limit on the amount of healing that you can do. But John does go out in the solarium and sit in his chair. They do have him up more than down. I can see where he could probably be encouraged to walk again. It would take a lot of work.

How does the medical staff respond with John?

Positively, very positively and favorably. It is really a team effort. The nurses are sensitive to John's needs. When they are about to change his dressing they will say, "Bev, we're doing John's feet," and I say, "Okay, I'll be right there." I noticed the difference in how they work with his feet. The little extra syringing, the little extra cleaning, the little extra, almost, love being poured into the care of his feet. They clean the area, making it especially clean for me to do the healing. John is getting a lot of care, you know, a lot of tender care. Changing the dressings is always a ritual. They really work together.

Is he as lucid with you now as before?

A very strange thing is happening lately. He is *more* lucid. The other day we actually had a conversation. "And how are *you?* I want to know how you are." I couldn't believe that he said it that way: that was just the way he said it. He said, "Never mind me. How are you?"

Sometimes I am on the ward to help with the feeding at lunchtime. John is usually around. Staff tease me, "Beverly, how do you rate? Look, he always knows you!" I just look at him and smile, and he'll look at me and smile. Sometimes he will say, "Oh, that's my girl."

And he told me he likes me. And he told me he loves me. He has told me that. He has actually said the words, "I love you." And he held my hand. I told him I loved him, too.

CASE 4: ROBIN J.

by Beverly Ryder

Robin J. was admitted four months ago to Cushing Hospital where she was placed on the Intensive Care Unit. She is eighty-nine years old and needs a lot of medical attention. She had been at a local community hospital with a history of multiple cerebrovascular accidents (CVAs) and reported problems with feeding. Tube feedings and intravenous feedings (IVs) had been considered.

The CH medical director reports that the daughter is not inclined toward heroic measures. Nursing staff notes that the patient does not have trouble swallowing but will refuse food occasionally. They find her alert and responsive to verbal commands. She is able to hold a glass of water when requested and to assist in her own movement. In the beginning, however, she did not eat by herself; she was always fed by somebody. Psychology reports indicate that she did not respond verbally nor did she respond to touch or follow a finger across her visual field. Psychology's impression is of chronic brain syndrome (CBS), severe. Physical therapy reports that the patient participated minimally in their efforts to evaluate her and is not a candidate for physical therapy treatment. Occupational therapy reports that the patient nods appropriately when addressed, and recreation therapy notes that the patient does establish eye contact and appears to understand. The medical director concurs and suggests that she has a "knowing look" even though she does not speak. He suggests that the patient could be manifesting global aphasia. She also had multiple decubitus, bilateral cataracts, and a history of urinary tract infection and hysterectomy.

These observations were offered during a patient care conference, during which time a number of suggestions were made in the hope of helping the patient to communicate more adequately. Because it did not appear necessary to feed through tube or IV, Robin J. was to be transferred to an extended care ward and her situation reviewed at this conference in a month.

I came to work with Robin when she was a new admission because of a referral that came out of the patient care conference. I would also like to mention that in addition to the conditions mentioned at the conference, Robin also was incontinent. She had a catheter but was incontinent of feces.

In my initial contact I felt that Robin had lots of potential and that she understood in her own way. The most striking thing about Robin was her eyes, so very beautiful, bright, and expressive. During the first meeting I sat very close to her and held her hand. I began to share with her what little knowledge that I have about strokes and how we could look for improvement. When I began to talk about technicalities she turned me right off. I realized that perhaps I was going a bit too far that way, so I gently patted her hand and said, "Don't worry, I won't push you. We will go slow and easy and work at your pace." With that, she responded and resumed eye contact, nodded to me, and smiled.

Our first few visits entailed a lot of touch and positive suggestions. I would tell her that she looked better and comment on her eyes. Sometimes I would just put my arm on her shoulder and say, "It's all right. Everything is all right." Once during the early visits her daughter came in and watched me working with the mother. The communication was crude at times, but the daughter was impressed, and she was very glad that her mother was getting this special kind of therapy. I explained a little of it to her, but she was very apprehensive about her mother's level of understanding. As a matter of fact, the daughter said that she was very much comforted by the thought that mother doesn't understand what's going on. I tried to explain tactfully to the daughter that this could be so, but that I believed that her mother might come to understand. She could get better in some ways, and even now she understood a little more than it might seem. This statement upset the daughter a little. She had come to the conclusion that her mother could no longer understand what was going on, yet she still was positive about my working with her.

I continued working with Robin in a very low-key way. I did not push her to do things, but I started noticing that as she talked, she would move her hands about and would want to touch things. I would comment on these actions and try to use them as a basis for strengthening her hands. "Perhaps you can learn to use your hands again," I would say when she did something with them on her own. If I was asking too much of her, she would let me know by turning me off. But if not, she would respond and nod appropriately.

How did you know she was turning you off? What did she do?

She would just look away, just turn her head and look away from me as if she were in another world. I sensed that this must be because of something that I was doing, so I learned from those experiences with her. I learned how to communicate with her and gradually, more and more, she allowed herself to do more. I picked up one of our orange sponge balls. She liked the brightness of it, you could tell. She started squeezing it to exercise her hands—she was still not talking but she was nodding more appropriately and smiling at one point.

I wondered if perhaps she would respond to music because she wasn't speaking. Maybe the side of the brain that was more in tune with music might spark something within her. Andrea came, then, and sang to her. She was very responsive to the music and really seemed to like it, though she still didn't talk or anything.

The next day she didn't remember Andrea but did recognize me, which I thought was a little encouraging. She would watch me as I walked in and smile at a distance, before I would have to get close to her to get eye contact. She seemed to be noticing more of the things that were around her. More and more, I felt a growing relationship, a loving give-and-take.

One day I asked her if Jean, her daughter, had been in. She nodded and looked extremely sad, tears in her eyes. I felt that this sadness had something to do with Jean. I put my arms around her and said, "You know, it must be hard for you. This must be so difficult, being in this kind of situation and knowing that everyone doesn't understand that perhaps *you* understand more than they think." And, you know, that was really amazing! She just looked at me and cuddled to me. That established some kind of a bond, a trusting bond. I felt that I was taking a gamble in talking to her this way, assuming something that I couldn't be sure of. But, when I left later, she was smiling and feeling happier.

I also began to sense that her trust was directed toward me, and that she was being rather secretive about it. She didn't want others to know. She was not ready to open up to the whole world.

This one day when I came into her area I saw a nurse whom I like very much. I feel she is a very good nurse. But she was very upset with Robin at that moment. "She is the dirtiest woman I have ever encountered," is what she said. I realized right away what was going on. Robin had probably had a bowel movement, and the nurse had a mess on her hands. I used to clean up patients a lot (years ago as attendant in a nursing home), and all kinds of things went through my head at that moment. I stood there a bit paralyzed while my mind was active. Then I literally backed out of that ward, just backed away. My thought was: "Robin mustn't see me." This was because Robin knows that I know that she understands.

Did the nurse say this within Robin's hearing?

Yes. But at this time the nurses were not all in agreement about Robin. Mostly they felt that she didn't understand, that she didn't have the kind of understanding that I thought she did. I went to my office and sat there for a good half hour or so, mulling it over in my mind: What am I going to do? How am I going to handle this? I decided I'd just have to go and see Robin. At least Robin doesn't have to feel that embarrassment and humiliation with me. I went in—and there she was, all curled up in a ball, and the tears were just falling out of her eyes, mucous was coming from her nose, and she was making little whimpering sounds, very quietly. It was terrible for her. I put the side rails down and kind of picked her up and held her. I kept talking to her, telling her that sometimes people didn't understand, but that I did understand.

Did you speak of the incident?

I didn't. I just couldn't do that. I said that sometimes people might hurt her feelings unintentionally, without meaning to do that, and that people do get upset. They have their bad days; we all do. I just tried to somehow justify or maybe neutralize—minimize—what had happened. I told her that she should feel good about herself. Robin cuddled herself to me and wept. I said it was all right. Things were going to get better. I was going to help her. I could see how she was going to do all sorts of wonderful things, and there were still wonderful things that were going to happen in the world. I spoke of the spring and coming to the garden and the renewal of good things. For a while she stayed quite sad. But then she would reach out and hold me, like holding on to something that was really solid. At that moment I felt a very strong commitment to her—that I would continue working with her no matter what.

I began working with Robin on her appetite. The nurses were having problems with her on that; she wasn't eating. I speculated to myself that the problem with her eating might have to do with her not being used to the catheter. Some people don't drink water or eat because of that problem. So I spent some extra special time with her, working on the eating problem.

How did you go about this?

I took my lunch. I went there during my lunch hour and began feeding her myself.

Did you feed her the hospital food?

Yes, and she ate better for me than she did for others. Sometimes I would bring coffee in. "We are going to have dinner together now." I made it a really nice experience, or I tried to. But sometimes there was a sadness there. But if I hadn't been there for a meal, I'd ask her if she had eaten. She would smile proudly and nod yes.

It was on December 12 that she spoke for the first time. I had always continued to speak to her as if she could speak. I'd say, for example, "How are you?" or "Did Jean come in today?" or something like that. Her daughter would come about once a week. So I went to Robin one day and said, as usual, "How are you?" And very clearly *she* said, "All right." I was shocked! So happy I was, so happy to hear this! When I tried to follow up on this talking, though, she hushed down to a whisper. She whispered in a secretive way and her eyes were darting all over the place.

I was so excited that I wanted to say something to a nurse. Robin's eyes darted around and they darted back to me, and she shook her head no. She was very frantic, really upset, and then angry at me. I immediately knew what it was. "I'm so sorry, Robin, I really am sorry; please forgive me." She shook her head no; she wasn't going to forgive me.

Can you make this a little clearer?

I said I was sorry because I was going to share her speaking with someone. The whole thing happened so fast! I told her that I didn't realize she didn't want others to know that she could talk. She realized that I really was sorry about being ready to tell the nurses, and she could forgive me for that. By the time I left she did end up forgiving me. I stayed there for quite a while, and it was all right. I assured her that I would keep this in confidence, a confidence between the two of us. I told her that when *she* felt like speaking to others, that I was sure she could. She accepted this. Gradually she did speak a word or two to other people. She was very selective about that.

Then I did things like reading cards to her. It was the Christmas season. I'd read her cards to her. Some of them were addressed to "Yolande." I discovered that this was another name some of her close people called her. However, she made it clear that she wanted me to call her Robin, not Yolande. I asked her if this was a sort of grandmother name for her, and she said this was correct. As I read the cards I said, "Do you know this person? Who is this?" And she would answer very clearly. She would say yes if she knew the person and no if she didn't. The ones she didn't know were generally friends of her daughter's. She so enjoyed the reading of the cards.

Her daughter came in and told me that she was pleased with her mother's progress. She hoped that I would continue working with her, but could I give her some advice as to a Christmas present. I couldn't think of anything right away. Then I explained to her about reading the cards. The daughter replied, "She doesn't remember anybody." I said that there were some she did remember, or at least she said she did. The daughter was skeptical about that. She was not ready to believe it. I didn't push it directly. Instead I suggested a photograph album for a gift, a family album. The daughter thought she wouldn't recognize anyone. I said that if she did get a family album for her, I would sit with Robin and go through the pictures; this would be something the daughter could do, too, if she wanted to.

The daughter did bring in a family album. This really surprised me because she had been so skeptical. She made up an album, and Christmas day I saw it and we went through it. I brought Robin a knitted shawl that tied around her shoulders, and I fed her Christmas dinner. She liked the shawl very much. She touched it and was very responsive to it. It was bright-bright colors, just what she likes. When we went through the pictures together, indeed, she did recognize people. She pointed herself out to me in one picture.

Little by little, we progressed. She began to do things for herself. It was after Christmas time. I had a few days' vacation planned, and I told her I would be away. It so happened that Lisa was nearby. Robin had observed Lisa and me together. We are together a lot on that ward working with various patients. As I was telling Robin that I would be away for a few days, there were tears in her eyes. She was very sad. I motioned to Lisa and said that she would be here. She's a lovely girl and she'll see you while I'm away. Robin almost angrily shook her head no and grabbed my hand. She just held my hand, patted my hand. However, I saw her again before the vacation, and she did seem to accept it.

Did she see Lisa?

Yes, Lisa did see her. When I returned I almost expected that she would be angry with me, but it wasn't like that at all. It was a wonderful reunion. She was very happy, held her arms out to me, and smiled. "Do you remember me?" I said, and yes, she nodded her head. We went through the picture book again. When we were through with the book I was just getting ready to close it up, and she moved her body toward me and kissed me on my cheek. So unexpected. It was the most beautiful, wonderful experience.

Do you recall the exact circumstances?

I was intent on what I was doing, closing up the book and getting ready to take my leave. And at that moment she moved her body toward me, with the effort that took, and kissed me on my cheek. I was touched by that and said, "Oh, Robin, thank you. That means so much to me." You know, I kissed her back. It was beautiful.

Then, in mid–January, there was a lot of progress from there on in. I continued to feed Robin daily. I also taught her how to feed herself. One triumph after another. She held the spoon and fed herself! She started to motion then for my notebook. I began to get the feeling that she wanted to write. I asked her if she would still talk. She replied with a lot of motioning and said two or three words at a time when I directed questions at her. But when she wanted to do something, she would motion more than talk. I would ask her, "Would you like to write?" She would nod yes. Sometimes she would say, "Yes."

So I handed her the pen. I tried to help her hold it. She was clumsy at first. I worked with her first in just holding the pen. Finally I could see that she felt comfortable holding the pen. I gave her the paper and she began to write. It was evident that she was writing *something*. When I looked at what she had written, it was little scribblings. She was very upset about that. I said, "Robin, isn't it wonderful how you are getting the feel of that pen! I bet it's been a long time since you have been able to hold a pen like that. Isn't it great!" I concentrated on that part of what she did to take away her feeling of disappointment. "After a while you are going to be able to write again. This is a good beginning. First things first, you know."

Robin responded very well to that. She smiled at me and the sadness immediately left. She did go from scribbling to making circles. I praised her for this and took these opportunities to explain a little about the connection between the brain and movements of our hands and bodies, and about brain damage. I said there were some problems with the connections, but that there was nothing really wrong with her. The body has its own healing process, and these things would clear up. She would be able to do more and more things. She was very responsive to this, and listened to any technicalities I brought in. It seemed to be a learning process for her about herself and her brain damage. It was incredible because she definitely was making progress at that time.

Another thing I want to mention here. It was during this time that she became continent—consistently. She began to do more little things for herself. Robin began to feed herself without my help. Because of this, they decided to move her. The daughter noticed this progress, too. Just before they moved her, they made her an activity tray. I explained to her that this was to help her manipulate her hands. The occupational therapy staff made the thing, but I worked with her on it. I explained to her that this was a kind of fun therapy for her hands, and she did enjoy it. One thing about Robin was that she loved praise. I'd praise her for the things she did and say how grand it must feel to be accomplishing them, and she would smile in acknowledgment.

At about this time I had another talk with her daughter. She said she had noticed a lot of progress and was very pleased that her mother seemed to be more aware. But you could see the daughter still had this apprehension, wondering about her mother's level of comprehension. I said that I thought Robin was understanding a lot more than she did before. Jean then went down to see her mother. I followed her, and was going by to see another patient when Robin suddenly turned from her daughter, looked at me, and reached out to take my hand in a sort of "hello." This shocked the daughter. She said, "My God, she really knows you, my God!" She was shaken up by this little incident. And then she said—with Robin sitting right there—"I wonder: do you think she knows me?" Up until then I didn't know that the daughter felt that her mother didn't know her. I said, "Oh, yes, I'm sure she knows you." Robin looked at me and at her and smiled as if to say, "See I'm still here—and I know." After this, I think the daughter felt less apprehensive.

How old is the daughter?

I'd say she was in her early fifties.

This is the end of January, and Robin got so much better that they decided to move her to Ward B. They asked me if I would mind telling Robin because she related so well to me. One of the nurses and I spent about half an hour explaining to Robin about the move. I was positive about it. I was telling her that we could do even more things together and that she would be able to get out and get to know the hospital. She was just kind of listening, with very little expression. I sensed her apprehension. I reassured Robin that I would still be working with her closely. That seemed to relax her a little, but when I got to the part about saying that where she had been was for the really sick and now she was better enough to move, Robin very clearly said, "I'm sick."

She said those words?

Yes, she did. She spoke them. And at that moment there was a nurse nearby to hear it. She said, "Beverly, tell Robin that we are going to miss her." Robin looked right at her, looked right at the nurse, and said, "Thank you."

It was marvelous. In a way, it was sad, too. But what was really sad was that Robin was moved in front of Charlotte W. (another patient).

What do you mean, "in front of Charlotte W."?

When they moved her, they put her in Ward B and directly in front of Charlotte W. One of Charlotte W.'s problems is jealousy. I work with her, and I'm hers exclusively—that's how she sees it. This became a very serious problem.

I never made this kind of request to Nursing before. I begged them to move Robin somewhere else. She said, "No, it would do Charlotte good to realize that you work with others." She felt very strongly about it. There was a little locking of horns about that. At that time I got sick myself and I couldn't see either Robin or Charlotte very much except for two or three times a week.

This situation disturbed me night and day. I would take it home with me. How am I going to solve this problem? Charlotte would say,

"I hate that crazy old lady!"—meaning Robin. And Robin could hear her say it. When Charlotte was going down to the bathroom or something like that, I'd take the opportunity to shower Robin with love and affection, but I saw the deterioration.

Instead of giving her a meal, they gave her that little yellow dish with mush in it. I could see the decline, and what was incredible about it was that she seemed to understand my dilemma! She'd look at me and pat my hand and smile as though saying, "It's okay." The kind of look she would give me, so understanding. It almost made it easy, you know, and I have to admit I feel a great deal of guilt about this.

When I came into the Monday morning meeting I heard that Robin was ill. There was a lot of flu going around. She wouldn't be going to ICU because there wasn't a bed there. So I went right to Robin from the meeting. It was one of the first times that I bypassed Charlotte. I had been seeing them together, but that time I just ran to Robin. She was very lethargic, having a difficult time breathing. I told her I was there. She didn't have too much of a response. I said things like, "You're going to get better," "We're going to do things together," "Oh, Robin, I really care so much for you," and that sort of thing. Still no response.

So I went then to the other side of the bed. I put my arm on her shoulders and leaned over to her ear. I said, "Robin, I love you so much." And with that, she turned her head, and just leaned against my shoulder, so I knew she was hearing me; I knew that she understood. She just leaned. It took all the effort she had. It was a very special moment.

When I went out—this is Ward B now where I've never done this— I said to the nurse, "If something serious comes up with Robin, please have me paged. She said, "Why, do you think something is going to happen?" I said, "I just have a feeling. I have this feeling. Please, please, have me paged." She promised she would. About two o'clock she did have me paged. She told me that Robin had gone to the ICU and that it was very serious. She was critical. When I got there, the daughter was with her and crying. The nurse was on one side of her and the daughter on the other. I walked over to the side where the nurse was, and she stepped back so I could get close to Robin. The nurse knew I had worked closely with Robin.

At first sight, it looked like she might be dead. She was so still. There wasn't much of anything going on; she was barely breathing.

I looked at the daughter, and she looked back as if she were happy to see me. The daughter continued crying, but you could tell that she felt more relieved and thanked me for coming.

I started to stroke Robin. "Here, Robin, I'm right here with you. It's me, Beverly." I saw her move her eyes, enough so her eyes could focus on mine. Then her eyes became kind of fixed. She took a breath. Her daughter looked over at the nurse, and was watching me with her and looking at the nurse. I asked if she had responded to anyone at all, and the nurse shook her head no. There was no response to anybody or anything. I kept stroking Robin while I was talking. Jean put her arm on the other side of Robin and was stroking her, too. I told Jean what had happened that morning, how at first she didn't respond but then did. I was just saying how Robin had leaned her head toward me so I knew that she did understand how much I loved her. And it was at that moment that Robin died. At that very moment. She was just looking at me.

How do you know she died at that moment?

Because she didn't take another breath, and she had just taken one. I didn't stop touching her, and I touched her for another fifteen or twenty minutes. I even talked to her, though I knew she was dead.

Did the daughter say anything?

The daughter realized that she had died at that moment, too, because she looked at me and I looked at her, and she was crying more. I started to cry, and I was saying, "Robin." The daughter said that Robin was so terrified of death. I don't know where I got the courage to do this, but I just looked at the daughter and I smiled, and I looked at Robin, and I gestured with my hand toward her, toward her face. I said, "She's not afraid. You can see, she's not afraid." And the daughter just looked at me and smiled. It was kind of a special moment.

Robin had looked unresponsive, didn't you say?

She looked very peaceful. But her eyes—there was a response when she moved her eyes toward my eyes when I told her I was there. As a matter of fact, the nurse said, "She was waiting for you both."

In the years ahead, the daughter will know how her mother died. She won't have to wonder or worry about that.

No. As a matter of fact, we hugged each other and cried in each other's arms.

You and Jean?

Yes, we did, and she just kept on thanking me, thanking me.

And the nurse?

The nurse put her arms around her, too. She put her arms around both of us and said, "It's all right. I know how close you feel." I was embarrassed because I was crying, and the nurse was saying, "Beverly, I understand. It's okay. You just cry."

All kinds of things were happening to me in my mind. I felt like Robin could hear. Then Dr. X. came in and we all stepped aside, and she used the stethoscope and pushed in her ribs and chest a few times. The doctor told the nurse that Robin was dead. The nurse said, "This is her daughter." Dr. X. turned to her and said, "I'm very sorry," and she walked out of the room. We all knew it was just sort of a formality, I guess, but I just felt so uncomfortable about it.

What made you feel uncomfortable about it?

It was so dehumanizing.

What was dehumanizing?

It was *automatic*. It was something that was automatic. The doctor probably had all kinds of feeling or maybe she didn't. It's just an automatic thing, to go in as if you were checking a computer or something, and she'd say it's not working, it's gone.

When she came in . . .

When she came in she didn't acknowledge anyone. She just walked to the patient and checked her out. I feel very uncomfortable talking about it. Then the daughter left, and I just kept stroking Robin. All kinds of things were going on inside my head, sort of communicating with her. After a while the nurse said, "Beverly, we have to wash up the body now." I wanted to help so I would know that it would be done with reverence, but then I couldn't, so I left.

This morning—today—the head nurse said that in all her years working with patients she had never seen anyone look as serene and peaceful as Robin did.

CASE 5: MATILDA D.

by Andrea George

Matilda D. was born in Germany, one of four children. Her two brothers are deceased, and her sister lives in another state. Matilda completed grammar school and later took night courses to further her education. In 1911 she married, but her husband was killed during World War I. At that time, Matilda was twenty-six years old and was unable to work full-time because she had two young daughters. She did factory work at home, as well as taking in ironing and doing others' housekeeping. In 1948 she came to this country to live with her daughter and her family. Later she was housekeeper to various families until she retired at age seventy. She maintained her apartment until she was seventy-five. At that time her arthritis became so painful that she moved in with her daughter in a community near this hospital. The stiffness in her fingers increased and spread to her shoulders and arms (it is now painful for her to be touched). She suffered a small stroke at age seventy-six and four years later underwent gall bladder surgery.

She can speak English but speaks German when she is excited or nervous. Matilda enjoys reading, classical music, and watching television occasionally. She is also a deeply religious woman. She was admitted to Cushing Hospital at age eighty-six.

Her medical history includes rheumatoid arthritis, anemia, malnutrition, and chronic brain syndrome.

I met Matilda D. about six months ago while Lisa was introducing me to some of the people she knew on the ward so I could get a feel of the hospital. Immediately I felt rapport with Matilda. I don't know what I felt, but I knew that I was drawn to her. When I was on that ward I would spend a lot of time playing my guitar, singing for Matilda. The first time I met Matilda she was lying down and was really arthritic. She'd been in pain for about ten years. She did sit up occasionally, but spent most of her time in bed. I played music for her, and she really loved it. Although Matilda couldn't sing she always told me that she was singing in her heart with me—and I could tell by her eyes that she was. Our relationship expanded, with music as its basis. I would sing German folk songs to her. I'd sing

Edelweiss just about every time that I met with her, and that small thing really made her feel good. It was just beautiful to see. And we'd talk about the mountains and the edelweiss flowering. She said she felt as though I was bringing her mountains from Germany into the hospital.

Another important part of our relationship was that we could communicate about nature and about God. We had those strong interests in common. She was a Christian Scientist, a very humble woman. Anytime I would give praise, she'd just shy away in a very cute way, as though she really wasn't beautiful and that I was absolutely ridiculous to think she was. But Matilda herself was always full of praise. She liked to tell me things about myself. For example, she would say that I had very deep lines in my hands and that God was with me all the time and that my hands were blessed—she could tell! Matilda would say this particularly when I had my hand on her head. Just her tone of voice and the way she would say a thousand, thousand thank you's when I would leave! and I'd *feel* a thousand, thousand thank you's.

Matilda thought that Lisa and I were spiritually identical. The fact that we looked alike to her and, I think, the fact that she trusted both of us became more and more important as she came closer to her *transition* because it was Lisa who was finally with her at the end.

I'll talk about Matilda chronologically now. I worked with her for two months and developed a trust relationship, a friendship. As we moved on toward Christmas-time, Matilda spent more and more time reclining on her bed. In fact, from December on, I never saw her sitting up. She had more days spent almost entirely in sleeping and more days in pain.

About a week before Christmas she told Lisa and me that she was dying. We talked to her about that, and we just helped her to feel that *it was okay*. We thanked her for sharing this feeling with us. It was a very important feeling, and we wanted the opportunity to help her feel comfortable with it. I asked her if she was afraid. She said no—very simply, "No, I'm not afraid at all." I thought that was really good. It gave us an open line of communication. We didn't need to work around corners; we could be honest together.

As I was leaving the hospital that day, I got this sensation. It was a kind of feeling that had the thought, "One or two." That is what came to me somehow. I thought, "Well, maybe that means that

Matilda has one or two weeks left." I continued to think about that. I waited on that hunch, and as it turned out, it was between one and two months. It was actually six weeks from then that she did make the transition. As time moved on we were aware that she was slowly getting weaker and coming closer to her transition. Matilda seemed as though she wasn't quite able to understand what to do about that—physically, I mean. Should she hang on and continue to bear the pain or what?

One day in January I asked Matilda if she had asked God to release her from her pain, had she asked God to help her let go of her body? Matilda looked at me as though to say, "No, but that's a heck of a good idea! I hadn't thought of that!" This seemed to be a breakthrough.

I felt she needed something else at this time. I brought an image to her. I said, "Matilda, you are really a beautiful white bird, and there's a beautiful white bird in your heart." It took her a little while to comprehend this image, but then she went with it. I said to her, "When you pray at night I want you to ask God to open the doors and let the bird fly. Let the bird go free." Matilda smiled. I think she appreciated that image and I could tell that it was helpful to her because on days when she had so much pain and weakness that I could get no positive response from her, I would return to the image. "Have you asked God about the white bird lately?" She'd look at me and smile, and her eyes would show me that this was an important part of her feelings, that it made her feel good, the thought of freedom from the great pain and weakness she was experiencing more and more. I'd see the nurses turn her over, and it was really sad to see her suffering so.

Matilda didn't like the fact that she was in a hospital. She once confided to me that she never thought she would end up in a place like this. She prayed for me that I never would. I told her that I understood, but that I would be with her to make it easier.

She was now starting to get sicker in a hurry, to deteriorate step by step. After about a week and a half she could hardly breathe. Her lungs were filling up. I couldn't reach into the nursing realm and say that she needed oxygen or anything else. I just had to do what I could, mentally and spiritually, with her. When she had been gasping for air for at least a two-day period, I brought music to her. Matilda was a pianist herself. She liked Mozart and Brahms, Bach, and Beethoven. I played a tape for her and said, "Matilda, this is Mozart."

She raised her eyebrows and had an expression of surprise and pleasure. Somehow Mozart had broken through all her pain and suffering. Other times, when I had my guitar with me, I'd ask Matilda if there was anything I could do to make her feel better. She'd just turn to me and say, "Andrea, give me your music." It was so special that this is what she wanted because this was all that I could do to help her bear her suffering. The music between us became more important as the words became less important. Finally, she was moved to the ICU and given oxygen and more attention.

I placed my tape recorder in Matilda's room along with tapes I made for her of Beethoven, flute and harpsichord music, an "Ave Maria," the Vienna Boys' Choir, and things like that. Every time I visited Matilda I played the tapes. It's interesting that as I played the tapes, the nurses became involved, too. I'd tell them to feel free to play the tapes anytime I wasn't there. I told them that Matilda loved music and I knew she could hear it. The nurses really got into that; they were good to Matilda.

I met her daughter at this point. The daughter was really astounded that her mother had music, that she had this attention, that there was someone there to love and to comfort her. The daughter appreciated this attention to her mother because she felt that Matilda was afraid. I was beginning to feel this, too. I think Matilda had come to some realization about death. In theory we say we are not afraid. But there is a point, you know, where you think, "Maybe what I've got is better than letting go and not knowing what I'll have." Matilda was also afraid for her daughter. I think she felt, "What will happen to my daughter when I'm gone?" She was feeling some *responsibility not to die*. Everyone here was paying attention to her. If she died she would be letting them all down.

In my meditations I would relate to her—mentally, on a subconscious level—I'd send her the message that this was all right to let go. She didn't have to hold onto these responsibilities forever.

One day her daughter got very upset. the "Ave Maria" was playing, and she (the daughter) was so moved that she couldn't stay any longer. I followed her out and stopped her. I knew it was important for me to talk to her at this point. I tried to explain where I felt Matilda was in her transition. I knew she could hear everything we were saying even though she wasn't speaking, and all she was responding to was pain when she was moved. You could see her wince and a tear come to her eye, but that was the only response. I asked her daughter to look for Matilda in her dreams. I told her I felt sure Matilda had been trying to communicate and square her relationship with her daughter so she could be released. It was her daughter who, in a way, was holding her from transition. The daughter was very surprised that I mentioned that. She told me, "I have been waking up in the middle of the night, and I feel my mother calling me. I hear her trying to talk to me." I told her, "That's okay. She *is* trying to talk to you, and part of your job at this time is to let her go. Just say, 'Okay, mom. I love you and it's okay for you to go. Don't stay on my account.' "

Three days after that, Matilda finally made the transition. I feel that this thing between her and her daughter was the key to the transition. Also, one other thing: this was the same night of the day that I talked to her daughter about this fact. I was standing by Matilda's bed, and I decided to sit down and meditate and send love to her in that way. During my meditation I had an image. I saw Matilda in a mountain meadow across from me. We were up, I would say, about 12,000 feet. We were sitting where the grass level was about to change to rock and snow. Then the scene changed. Matilda showed me that she was trying to walk up the side of the cliff where there was all rock and snow. She had to climb this summit, and she couldn't do it. She kept slipping back and falling—and then it flashed back again and she was sitting in front of me. This was her predicament. She could find no way to get further in her climb. I felt like I was witnessing a guidance that came to her. As soon as she was back sitting opposite me again, the white bird appeared between us. This white bird was a recurring image in her transition, so it's important. The guidance that came to her—through me, or whatever—was that she should feel herself within the heart of the white bird. She should go with the bird, and the bird would take her beyond the earth. This earth-bound existence could take her no further. She would need another mode of transportation, so to speak. Matilda was to become the heart of the white bird and just fly and fly and fly until she couldn't feel her wings anymore. Pretty soon, then, the bird's heart— which was really *her* heart—would be God's. Then it would be okay because she would have found her road, her way of traveling. In this image she smiled at me and flew off, and the meditation was over.

I stayed with her a while longer that night and saw her the next day. Lisa and Beverly also saw her with me then. That was really beautiful because we, the three of us, surrounded her, and I felt that our energies really blanketed her with love and with the comfort and energy I think a person needs during that transition, especially when their life has been one of such suffering.

There was a time when all three of you were together with her?

Yes, the day before her final transition. Her daughter walked in, and you could feel the brain activity in Matilda's head. She was very aware at that point, so I brought her a poster, a huge poster, of the Alpine mountains. It was a picture that gave strength to the atmosphere. It reached the subconscious mind of everyone present, including Matilda and her daughter. This kind of atmosphere was much needed at the moment, along with the music and the love and support she was getting. It was all special and rightfully so, a beautiful way to make the transition.

I knew on the Thursday that she passed away that I wouldn't see her again. I was leaving to go to Wisconsin that evening, and I said goodbye to her. I told Matilda that God would be with her and my love would also be with her. She finally made her transition that evening when Lisa was with her.

I felt that my communication with Matilda was complete. From my mind to her mind was so simple. With some people, there are so many obstructions that you have to find out what they are and wade through them. But with Matilda it was simple. Every time I would leave her bedside I'd always know whether she was communicating or not. I would tell her that I was leaving my blanket of love, the beautiful purple blanket of love, and that it would stay with her and protect her until I came back again. When we meditated together the laying-on-of-hands wasn't that essential. I would always just sit and meditate, and this would bring her into the realm of our thoughts or a realm of universal mind. The meditation brought her places that were comforting and surrounded her with light and love.

The white bird: can you recall, first of all, why you presented her with any images at that time, and why the white bird in particular? Had this image come to you before? Had you used it before?

It was the first time I had ever used that image in a situation where a person was dying. I have never been that close in relationship with someone who was dying, and this was my first close relationship at Cushing Hospital, where I had begun as a volunteer. I don't know what happened; it was just a feeling I got; the image came to my mind and I knew I had to tell her about it; it was good for her and it was the way for her to release.

The white bird grew out of the situation, then; you hadn't been carrying it around in a cage? Go back to your first meeting with Matilda. Why did you see her in the first place? What goals or objectives did you have at the start?

It would be difficult to say what the goals were because I was just volunteering here as a healer and I know my goal was to heal, in all situations. I don't always have to ask myself why or how or what the purpose is. The purpose is always to heal. As an instrument of that healing energy, as an instrument of God, I know that everything I do is healing. I don't have to question my actions because I know that they always are the right actions. I know that I was what Matilda needed in this situation. I knew that my words would be right for her, that my intentions were always to soothe her and to help her cope with her pain and, as the issue came up, eventually to cope with her own death.

Unlike a traditional therapeutic approach, you aren't saying that "My goal is to heal Symptom A, solve Problem B, or anything of that nature." Your intention is simply to heal. That verb does not really need a noun. Is that what you mean? For instance, suppose that an outsider had been on the scene. This person saw you with Matilda but had no other information about what you were doing and why. What would this person actually have seen you doing? I am emphasizing the observer's direct observations—not what you felt or thought you were doing, but what another person could actually see. Let's take the first few times you saw Matilda before she became so very sick and weak.

They would have heard me playing my guitar, sitting on the bed opposite her, singing to her, laughing with her, talking and telling stories. Her telling me a story and kissing my cheek. Or my hand on her head. Most often I had my hand on her head. Every now and then your observer might sneak up on me with my eyes shut and Matilda sleeping, that sort of thing. Or me getting a Dixie cup of water, trying to find a straw from which she could drink, trying to find a nurse to change her position in bed. At that time the nurses may not have known for sure who I was. They would see me "hanging around" and being with Matilda. I feel more comfortable when they think I'm a relative because then they can't try and criticize what I'm doing. If I'm her granddaughter or something I have a right to be there with my hand on her head, laughing and joking.

Later on, Matilda became weaker and less responsive. Tell me what you actually did from an outsider's point of view, but also what you felt, what was going on inside you. I'm asking you to be true to your own experience, whatever it was. But you might also wander a little to explain what you thought was happening as well as your direct experience of what really was happening.

When she was moved to the ICU I was there a lot of the time. The nurses left me alone because, in a way, they were leaving Matilda alone, too. They knew she was dying. I really don't know if this gave them a feeling of discomfort or not. It didn't bother me, and they seemed to figure that if somebody wanted to stay with her, well, that's less time that they have to spend in a room with a woman who is dying. This is the attitude I felt from the nursing staff. Some of the nurses on Ward A told me, "Oh, it would be a blessing if she died." This seemed to carry another message: my time there was pretty much unnecessary—don't pray for her to live or anything like that. My attitude in response was, "That's cool. I'm not praying for her to live; don't worry about that." Not that they even suspected me of praying! But somehow they suspected that I wanted her to live or something! At one point I asked if her lungs would continue to fill up. The nurse assured me that they would. This was a common symptom of a patient who is about to die. But then her lungs didn't continue to fill up; they dried out some, and the breathing was more and more relaxed, and you couldn't hear anymore of that liquid sound. When a nurse told me this lung filling up was a common thing, I said it didn't *have* to be. I'm a psychic healer, and I made sure that the lung consistently drained, and that wasn't one of her problems. She didn't need that one!

You found out that she had a specific distress. Did you pray or meditate then specifically to keep her lungs dry and healthy?

A very short period of time was spent clearing the lungs out. It didn't take very much time to make sure that they were clear. I concentrated on it once when I was in the hospital, but mostly by meditating when I was at home. It didn't make much difference whether I was meditating with her at the hospital or by myself at home.

After Matilda died, did she appear to you in any way, any dreams or feelings?

Yes, actually, that Thursday. I had already flown to Wisconsin. I knew there was a great possibility that I wouldn't see her again in the hospital. In the few days I was away, when I would think of Matilda, I'd ask, "Where are you, Matilda?" One time when I asked this question I saw a flock of birds on the side of the road and they all flew up at once. There was one white bird among them. I said, "Okay, that's a good hint." The next day I was in a church at a wedding. My seat was in a pew with the only stained glass window. This window picture had a white bird with a green laurel in its mouth, and I *knew.*

Here is a low-down, mean question for you: how would you know if you were ever wrong? I am not talking about your good will, your intention to heal and comfort. What I am talking about now is what might be called your technique, your approach. Skillful therapists of all schools ask questions of themselves. Did I handle this situation right? Did I understand what was happening? Could I have done better? But you—you are always right! How could you recognize it if you were wrong? How do you evaluate and improve? As you can see, I am importing a whole different frame of reference from the one you have been using, a more traditional, professional, and scientific frame of reference. Deal with it.

I will. You have to remember that this is the first case I have been involved in at this hospital, let alone the first person I have seen die. I didn't have any certainty at all in how to deal with a dying patient. I had no frame of reference. I'd never done it before. I only knew Matilda and I only knew that I cared and that I loved her. And I knew she was in need when she was in need—even if I didn't know what she was in need of. I felt she needed my simply being there and praying for all that is best and highest for Matilda. To come to her at that point—maybe that was the best I could do!

There were times, sure, when I was afraid. I knew she needed to be moved. I knew there was no way in hell that we were going to get a nurse right then and there. She wanted to move a little, and she'd ask me to give her a little push from the back. I didn't want to push her. Her body is tiny and arthritic and I didn't want to hurt her. There is no way that I would want to inflict pain on this woman.

But I'd push. And then afterwards I would apologize and say, "I hope I didn't hurt you. If I ever hurt you, please forgive me." She understood.

I have to speak from a spiritual point of view. Sometimes I felt guided, that our relationship was guided. This was even more important for Matilda, as I realized at the time. Things happen for a purpose, and people come together for a purpose. I just felt that I went with the flow of how it felt. I tried to be open-minded, to keep my intuition flowing. I didn't go out on a limb or anything. I didn't feel like I was taking chances or anything. I always just did what was most logical.

Is that what you wanted?

Was that the kind of answer I expected? No. But you did get something across. You saw yourself as feeling, thinking, and acting in a natural and logical way. As long as you felt right about yourself within the situation, you felt that whatever you did was right, too. This approach has a kind of verification strategy, but it is private, subjective, difficult to get out and examine.

I don't doubt at all that you felt love for Matilda and communicated it in some way. But how was it possible for you to fall in love with an old lady so quickly? What was it that happened?

I asked myself that. When I first came to Cushing I wondered about this place as I walked through it. There isn't a lot of obvious beauty here, but you look a little deeper, through the decrepit old bodies, and you see a beautiful self that has been alive not only for an entire lifetime, giving and sharing, but perhaps other lifetimes. There's a whole feeling of that universal love in the situation. That's all I know. Matilda, in particular, could relate to me and that made it easier for me to relate to her.

You had a relationship with Matilda. So did her daughter. Would you say something more about these relationships, taking into account the possibility that the daughter might have been puzzled or offended by somebody else suddenly having a close relationship with he mother? You have said some things that are relevant to this question. Do you have anything to add?

A great deal to add, and that's an important issue. The first time I met her daughter she was absolutely unaware that I had already been working with her mother for three months. I explained some of the things that I did, and how I felt about Matilda. It was a pretty simple conversation. I also gave her my home phone number and asked her to call if she ever needed me for any reason. I felt that she was very touched and pleased. She was comforted and relieved. I guess I was lucky in this first situation of mine that she felt that way. Otherwise, maybe I would have been thrown for a loss. But it worked out well, and she called me after that and told me how she had been so impressed with what we are doing with her mother. She thanked me and said, "You know, it would be nice if there were an 'Ave Maria' for her to hear." The next time the daughter walked into the room, "Ave Maria" was playing, her mother was lying in bed, and she couldn't handle it. At first I was afraid—had I flipped her out? She thought perhaps her mother was dead. Then she started to cry. The daughter is a very emotional German woman. She started walking out, and I knew that I had to go after her, and that's when I talked to her about the dream. What was really happening was that she wasn't offended in any way. She was deeply touched, and she was so grateful that her mother was being given the surroundings and love that she truly deserved. She had worked hard all her life and given a great deal. Music was the most important gift I could have given her mother. You can't question the fact that things happen for reason. Why was I drawn to Matilda?

There would be times when I'd be standing at her bed and asking for whatever God would have done. I wouldn't ask that Matilda be taken. I wouldn't ask that she be made whole again. In terms of her body, it's not up to me to make choices for her; it's up to God. But many times, with my hands upon her, in particular the Tuesday or Wednesday before she passed away, incredible words would come through my mind to her mind. As though a drop of water were raining on the ocean, it would come and then pass away. They were words that I couldn't hold on to. They weren't meant for me. They were only directed through me.

So you felt that you were a vehicle or agency for communicating something valuable to Matilda. When you would leave Matilda after having been with her for a while, did you feel drained emotionally, or how did you feel yourself?

I forgot one very important thing. It was one time, just after the white bird had come up, and Matilda was not suffering too much and could still communicate and joke. She said, "Andrea, I forgot to tell you. Last week, one night, I saw you in my dream." I was thrilled by this because healing can be done on a soul level, as far as I believe. I asked what I was doing in her dream. She said, "You were standing here just like this; we were talking." Then Matilda got a special look in her eyes and said in her own little way, "You know, Andrea, *this is mind reading!*" I laughed and said, "I know— it is beautiful, isn't it!" And when I left the hospital that night there were tears in my eyes. I was so impressed with the fact that the connection was so total that I walked into the house and wrote a poem for Matilda.

I asked a question a few minutes ago, and now I'm wondering whether or not I've heard the answer. When you would leave Matilda after a session, did you go away with a sense of having been emotionally drained? No. That wasn't it at all. What word would you use then, what describes the way you felt?

Unification.

CASE 6: LEONARD R.

by Lisa B. Hathaway

Leonard R. was born in Lithuania, one of five children. He attended only night schools and worked in a mill. His immediate family includes his wife, son, and daughter.

Basically in good health all of his life, Mr. R. fell from a ladder at age ninety-one. He fractured his jaw in this accident and was treated for six days in the geriatric service of a university hospital. After returning home, he showed signs of forgetfulness and was at times incontinent of urine. Despite these problems, he continued to work in his garden and carry out his customary daily routines. However, his wife—herself only two years his junior and suffering from a heart condition—found it difficult to care for him at home. He was in his ninety-first year when admitted to Cushing Hospital.

Medical history at time of admission included, in order of significance: chronic brain syndrome, right inguino-scrotal-reducible hernia; benign prostatic hypertrophy; exogenous; deafness, partial, bilateral; chronic stasis dermitis of left leg; phlebitis of left leg (history).

Leonard R. was brought to Cushing without his knowledge. His daughter and wife put him in the car and said, "We're going to take you for a ride." When they arrived here, he walked into Cushing. The supervisors made him comfortable, and he said, "Where are we? What are we doing here?" The family said, "You're going to be here a few days." The nursing supervisor looked at everybody and said, "You mean he doesn't know?" They shrugged.

I saw him very soon after he came in, but didn't see him again, to really start working, for another six days. My intention was to be honest with him no matter how much it hurt. That was the only way we could possibly cope with the situation. I wanted to comfort, to help him adjust, and to be his strength here, somebody he could rely on.

I went to see him primarily because he was restless, looking around for his wife. His family brought him in without preparing him, and it was hard for him to make sense of the situation. There was an immediate bond between us, even though he was speaking about 98 percent Lithuanian or Polish. I don't know the difference between these two languages, and he speaks five languages altogether. He is a very smart man. He did slip a little English in. For example, when he met me, he said, "You look like my daughter." He did not mean my looks as such but something about me. He immediately gave me a kiss on one cheek and a kiss on the other cheek, and then a hug. He was so glad to see me.

I didn't have to explain why I was there. The important thing is that I *was* there and he needed somebody, so I just helped him in any way that I could. They had to keep him restrained because they were afraid of his running away. This man could walk. He had a cane, and he would try to get in and out of all the doors and windows, while at the same time having a heck of a time trying to figure out what was going on.

There was also a management problem. There was a note on him saying that he was disturbing other patients and was slightly resistant to p.m. care. He would not speak English on a particular shift, and he didn't seem to understand simple commands. He had no complaints and was cooperative but confused, and he often looked for his wife.

I knew I wanted to work with him, but it took six days to adjust my schedule. When I worked with him he was relaxed. He had a beautiful big smile and you just wanted to give him a big hug all the time. He was such a good man, so affectionate. He always greeted me with a kiss. He knew my name, but often said, "Oh, you are like my daughter!" When he saw me his eyes lit up and his arms opened up wide, "Oh, you come to see me." "Sure, I did—do you remember my name?" "Yeah—Lisa!" He read my name tag and commented on what small print it had, and he also read newspapers and whatever else was around.

I let the staff know how alert he had been, how he tended a garden last summer, how he read the newspaper every day, and how he would take his lawnmower apart and put it back together. Well, his daughter said he didn't always put it back together right, but he certainly enjoyed tinkering with it. I acquainted the staff with these things about him because I didn't want them to see him too much as a confused person. I was afraid that when his behavior didn't seem to make much sense and he might be hard to manage, they might turn to medication. So I left a note on the cardex: "Page me if he gets agitated."

Did they page you?

Seven times! It seemed like even more, every time I turned around. He wanted to go home with the day shift, and nobody could go home because he was just latching on to them. He was also still looking around for his wife. I stayed with him for a couple of hours. He talked about many things, initiating a lot of the conversation. He gave me his impressions of the various attendants on the ward, and then told me of an incident with his mother long ago. He had eaten nine bananas at one time, and his mother got angry at him until he explained that he just loved bananas. I told him that I would bring in some. He was agitated during the early part of this conversation, but then he gave me a kiss on the cheek and a hug and remembered who I was. When I left him finally on that occasion, he was a lot calmer and was reading a magazine.

I went to the nurses' office and was writing a note on the chart when all of a sudden I had the strangest feeling come over me. I didn't know what was wrong, or what I was looking for, but I ran out of the office. Instead of running to where I had left Leonard, I ran toward the corridor. I ran into Charlie (another patient) and he said, "That man went that way! Outside! Outside!" So I ran outside, and there was Leonard. He had just stopped a girl who was driving away from Cushing. He walked in front of the car and it slowed down, and she got out and was holding him there. I went to Leonard and brought him back. It was strange because I would have wasted a lot of time if I had gone back to see him instead of starting right down the corridor. That's the only time I had that feeling. It was so fast. I didn't question it. I just acted on it.

Had Leonard said or done anything to suggest he might be heading out?

Nothing. He was just quietly reading his newspaper, and I was just sitting in the office. There were no nurses around right at that minute, and I was just writing on the chart, and I left my pocketbook and everything and just ran when that feeling came over me. I told Charlie later that he had done a lot of good—and he was so proud of himself. He (Charlie) is really psychic himself, so I'm not surprised that he was standing there to tell me where to go.

I was paged to the ward again and found Leonard standing behind a chair in the solarium on the other side of the ward, very uptight, very resistive. His attitude seemed to be, "I've got to get out of here. What's going on? Nobody touch me!" I decided that instead of approaching him directly I would just go in and sit in the chair. I watched him pace back and forth for a while and resist everybody else. I asked the others to leave. I just sat there and kind of looked at my hands. Finally I said, "Hi, Leonard." He said, "Don't! Don't say 'Hi' to me!" I said, "Okay, I'm not going to talk." I sat there for a good long time. After a while I said to him, very gently, that a lot of people loved him and that he was just going through a really hard transition. "It depends on how you want to do it. It's up to you. You can tear everybody down with you, or you can really try to understand what's going on—but I know you don't want to hurt your family."

Are those the words you used to talk to him?

Yes. He listened. Then while I sat there quietly, he sat down next to me. This was a good development because he had been keeping himself behind the chair where people would have a hard time getting to him. When he sat down I told him, "You don't have to like me, but please don't decide to hate me so soon!" I just felt strongly that I should say that. Then Leonard started talking, saying, "Oh, I didn't mean to do that," and so on. He settled down then. No more pages for the rest of the day!

Leonard did not have a very good idea of where he was. His bed was in the ward area, and it was not unusual for one confused old man to land in another one's bed. The beds usually have name tags, but they are small. I did him a really bright and crazy design in a color that he loved. It said LEONARD R. in big letters. I thought he'd grumble, "What's this?" but he said, "Oh, that's really nice." He was pleased with the design and the colors and, I think, pleased that somebody had made something special just for him.

At this time his daughter, an RN, had called from out of state, saying that she doubted her mother was planning to visit the patient in the near future. She really didn't want to have anything to do with him at this point for whatever reasons.

Leonard was still very agitated at times. He was not easy for the staff to manage. Once he struck an LPN on the mouth. The ward would page me and I would help Leonard quiet down. He would be relaxed and drifting off to sleep when I left.

This is still within a few days after admission?

Yes. It felt as though he was the only person I was really working with for a while because the need was there. I tried to make his life in the hospital richer and happier. It was getting into the Christmas season, so I brought Leonard to the recreation hall where a choir was singing. He loved it and the other activities going on there. He was a great socializer. He greeted everybody and started a lot of conversations. This was also good for the staff of his ward. They were saying, "You know, we can't take our eye off him for a moment," and this was an extra burden to them. But I knew Leonard could socialize because he was relating so well to me, so I took him off for many of the holiday activities and he was great, beautiful. It happened to be a perfect timing for his admission because of all the Christmas activity. People are usually happier and more vibrant at this time of the year, and I thought that Leonard could become a part of this, and he did.

There was a part of Leonard's personality that made it difficult for some staff to relate to him. He is very meticulous about everything he does. You can see it in the way he puts on his glasses, in everything. Some people don't have patience with that. And there was another problem. Leonard used to enjoy working with his hands, building things: for example, sleds. I tried to interest him in occupational therapy, but they evaluated him as having too short an attention span. They didn't think he knew what was going on and couldn't handle a project. I was hoping he could get into gardening or woodworking or something like that.

I brought him into occupational therapy one time and he took the hammer and started pounding away at different things. He was having a good time, even though he wasn't really making anything at that point. I thought this was a good beginning, that he was in a creative frame of mind, as though he was thinking, "What can I do with this?" Occupational Therapy didn't see it that way, though. I pushed one of the staff on this, and she said, "He is more interested in getting out the door than anything else." I asked when she had evaluated him. "Well, the first day he arrived!" I replied, "Well, it's been a couple of weeks since then," and she got kind of upset. I really pressed the point, though, because I felt that Leonard had a lot of things going for him and I wanted him to have every opportunity while he was still "hot" and interested.

Weekends were bad for Leonard. He was more assaultive and agitated. He couldn't wait to tell me that he had company for a half-day on Saturday because his daughter had come in. He was always trying to get me or Andrea to visit his home with him, to see his wife and his house and everything that was part of his life. It was a big thing in his mind for me to see these things.

I did ask the librarian to bring him some large print books from the book cart because he did love to read. I brought newspapers to him, but the nurses at first thought he wasn't really reading them. They thought the newspaper was just something he looked at and put down, but he really could read, and the nurses noticed this two months later. "This guy can read!" one of the nurses said. "You know, I think you should bring in some books for him." I said, "Really, what makes you think he can read?" "Well," she said, "He read the sign on the medicine door, Do Not Enter While Pouring Meds, and then he read something off from my journal. I said, "Yeah, I know; that's kind of neat, isn't it?" She agreed and said they would get newspapers for him regularly. It made me feel good that nursing appreciated more of what Leonard had going for him. We brought books to him — the Readers Digest large print editions — and he read them. When I brought the books to him, Leonard told me how important education was and then went on to speak for quite a while about his children and grandchildren. He spoke in a very positive way about them, no grudges or hard feelings.

Within eight days after I started working with Leonard, he was no longer searching for exit doors or unlocked windows, which really pleased me. Nursing was relieved about this change in his behavior. He was responding well to all. Four days before Christmas, I thought, "Leonard has really got it made." So I took a week's vacation. I came back to find that total disaster had hit for the week I was gone. He had become very agitated and aggressive. He didn't want anyone near him, didn't want to take his meds. He had a lot of problems. And wouldn't you know — they moved him to another ward while I was gone. He became disoriented all over again and went back to speaking Lithuanian, and the ward was having lots of problems.

He did wander off again. They had to call the state police, but it turned out that he had just wandered to the empty side of 309 and was sitting there quietly by himself. He felt really proud that he had managed to have a half-day by himself, a little cubbyhole where he could sit and meditate or whatever. But Leonard was still combative. He'd refuse to go to bed, take medications, anything. They said he was confused; he'd wander off if he wasn't closely supervised. I didn't find that true in my relationship with Leonard. When I had worked with him we would go to Times Square,[3] and take a right turn to get there. One day he stopped me. I said, "What's wrong, Leonard?" And he said, "We always go to the right. Let's go to the left this time." I thought it was kind of neat for him to say that. He might have been old and sick, but he liked trying something new.

When he went to the new ward he had a lot of problems and they put him on more medication, Thorazine.

What do you mean by "a lot of problems"?

They had to watch him every second. They had to keep him posied in a chair because he was agitated and trying to walk around. They took his cane away because he pointed it at some of the staff as if to say, "You stay away from me!" So when he walked, now it was more difficult for him. He wanted a little bit of that freedom that we shared together.

So I came back and kept telling him that I didn't leave him, didn't abandon him; I had just been on vacation. I had told him this before I left for vacation, but now I had to say it all over again. We took our usual walk, then, though I was feeling guilty for having been away. I explained where I had been and what was happening with him, why he was on another ward, why it was much better for him. At that moment a woman passed by, and tears came to his eyes. I said, "What's the matter?" "She looks and dresses like my wife." George L. (case 8) was with me while this was taking place, and saying, "It's okay, buddy." This was a very touching thing. Leonard straightened up and said, "Okay." One old man had helped the other get hold of himself.

Within a day after I had gotten back, the staff said Leonard was quiet and cooperative. Well, he did turn the shower on one day and took the hose and sprayed it all over walls, ceilings, floors, and into the laundry cart. They weren't too happy about that one. But Leonard, he had a blast! He was soaking wet but having a great time.

One night we were coming back from the recreation hall where we had seen a movie. Leonard says, "You know what, every Thursday

3. The central area of Cushing Hospital where the canteen, recreational therapy, patient's library and public people-watching space are located.

night I always used to kiss my mother and father goodnight." And this was a Thursday night. It was interesting that he just knew his own time and space in a certain way. He was really oriented to what was going on.

At this point he could ambulate in the ward area with no problems whatsoever. He was speaking more and more English to the staff, but this didn't mean that he was free from problems. He was still difficult to manage on weekends, especially if his family came in. His wife had come in once or twice, but that seemed to initiate that "I-want-to-go-home" feeling. When his family was around Leonard seemed to realize more sharply that he was not at home and that was where he really wanted to be. In general, though, the staff noted that he appeared to be settling down, and had had no night medication for three nights, sleeping well. The staff said he was doing fine because he was not a behavior problem, not that he was doing perfectly fine. After ten weeks he still felt something of the first shock of, "Hey, I'm really here!" I explained to him that his wife loves him very much but doesn't have the stamina to care for both of them. I told him what a hard decision she had to make to bring him here, and that she might have some trouble in facing him. He understood this and wanted to meet his wife whenever she could come into see him.

I continued with Leonard even though all the reports said he was in a good mood, talkative, ambulatory, no problems. Just because he was not acting out didn't mean that everything was all right. He had things to share and needed somebody to share them with. Leonard told me, "I will die soon." "Why?" I asked. "Because before, I could sleep, eat, garden, walk around when I want to; now, no more." We had a really long conversation about that. He knew the options he had. He said that this was like so much else that had been in his life; you just have to go through some difficult situations and do the best you can. I told him I knew how hard it was for him, that he had lost all that he had at home and hard to start over again here. "Hang onto your memory," I told him. "You still have your family and they love you. They will come in to see you, and I will help you rekindle some of those good feelings here at Cushing."

Leonard felt better after we talked about these things for a long time. When I was ready to leave, he said, "When you come back to me, you say to me, 'Leonard, are you still alive?'" The way he said this was humorous; he meant for it to be funny. He felt secure enough to let me go. It wasn't the "I-want-to-go-with-you" thing, which it had been in the beginning. He knew I was coming back. He did continue to get discouraged, though. He would say, "I have nothing here. I have no life here—but when you come, it's okay." I introduced Leonard to Marianne T. who is a volunteer, an incredible lady. I knew I couldn't hang in there much longer with him and still care for other patients, too. I wanted him to have somebody else as a support.

I did meet with Leonard's daughter. We sat by ourselves and talked. I told her what a tremendous adjustment he had made after his abrupt admission. She seemed surprised. She hadn't thought there was anything wrong with his admission. I told her, "This man is 100 percent with it. You have to recognize what he's capable of. He surpasses so many people of his age." The daughter was surprised to hear this. I told her that there were still adjustments to be made. "Well, he's doing fine," she said. I agreed, but pointed out that he still had things to work out and also needed interesting things to occupy his time. I asked her about the things Leonard was interested in. She thought that he would have been a genius if he had had the right schooling. He was always creating things, fancy sleds and toys for the kids, and always trying to invent new ways and better things. She pointed out that he had learned five languages without any schooling. "He just did everything on his own." She thought he would have a hard time if he couldn't go around puttering with things, putting machines together, gardening. We had been trying to find interesting things for him to do, but it remained a problem.

I often told Leonard how much he had going for him. "You have such great qualities, Leonard, and I can't stand to see anything so good go to waste. I want to help you to use those qualities you have and your strength." I would praise his stamina when he'd hold a cup of tea, and about his control when he'd spread butter on his bread, from corner to corner, ever so nicely and evenly. Staff who were trying to give him his p.m. care sometimes were frustrated by his slow and meticulous ways. He'd have to wash his glasses in a certain way, and they just wanted to get him quickly washed and into bed, while he wanted to do it himself, nice and slow.

Despite all these differences and problems, Leonard and the staff came to care for each other. The 7 to 3:30 shift, for example, wrote on the chart, "Patient usually cooperative and lovable." I discussed with the nurses the idea of building a sort of miniature greenhouse for Leonard, a shelf where plants could be brought in and he could tend them, and maybe later on the screened-in porch where he could grow tomatoes. Nursing pushed for this, and maintenance came down the other day and measured for the shelf.

I hated to stop working with Leonard. I wanted to keep seeing him, but not quite so often. He did have his relationship with that terrific volunteer, and I would kind of keep in there, but I had to take on other patients, too. Leonard was a fine, gentle, good man, and I really learned a lot from him.

Addendum

During one of our last sessions together, he asked me, "What do you think? Am I going to be here ... maybe two, three years?" I said, "I'm afraid so, Leonard, I'm afraid so ... at least that long." He looked at me for a moment, then said, "Well ... okay! That's all right." Then we hugged.

Two weeks later, when therapy had been discontinued, I felt strongly that I should see him. I kept trying to see Leonard all day long, but obstacles steadily formed in my path, small emergencies here and there. This same day I had received two different transcripts of his case. At home that evening I sat down and spent hours reading the transcripts and reminiscing of our time together. Then, at 12:05, my random thoughts quickly focused into an overwhelming sensation of love and good will for Leonard. I felt warm and secure, at peace. A smile appeared, and I found my eyes filling with tears of joy. I thought perhaps Leonard had included me in one of his dreams, so I sent him love and freedom from all negations in the form of an absent healing. This high state of being continued until 12:45 a.m., and then it stopped. The release came, and I fell asleep.

The next morning I learned that Leonard had had a slight fever and unexpectedly died during the night. I then surprised the nurse by telling her the approximate time of death. He was found dead at 12:45 a.m. I felt that he died at 12:05. Nobody knows for sure.

One of the attendants who knew how close Leonard and I were went through his belongings and returned the bright design I had done for him. She felt that I should have it.

CASE 7: HELEN C.

by Beverly Ryder and Judy Doran

This woman was born eighty-seven years ago in a neighboring community where she grew up, completed high school, worked a while, married, and had one daughter. Ruth gradually withdrew from her social life to dedicate herself to bringing up her daughter, who had some physical problems. They were quite devoted to each other. Twelve years ago, the daughter contracted pneumonia and died. Helen had a very difficult time accepting her death. She and her husband subsequently moved into apartments for the elderly. Later they were both admitted to a nursing home. Their relationship there was reported to be problematic, and they were separated and gradually lost contact with each other. She was later admitted to a local general hospital because she had become very weak and dehydrated. Her husband died of pneumonia, but as far as we know she has not been told of his death, at the request of her niece.

By the time she entered CH, Helen had many physical problems, with chronic brain syndrome the most basic. Prior to admission, she had had surgery for bilateral cataracts.

Beverly Ryder's Account

The first time I saw Helen she was curled up in her bed, a woman with snow-white hair and a foggy film over her blue eyes, perhaps related to her cataract surgery. There was something about her that got to me, her being curled up and just lying there.

I went over to her and put my head sideways to try to follow her gaze. Our eyes finally met. I put my arm around her shoulder and told her that my name was Beverly, that I'd come around to visit with her this evening and hoped she wouldn't mind. She said, "That's all right; that's fine." I asked how she was feeling, and she "guessed" that she was all right. There was a moment of silence— and then she began to count: "One, two, three; seven, eight, nine," counting in sequences of three. This turned out to be something she does characteristically. I wonder if it's an attempt to hold onto something—to her own mind, to be logical and orderly. I'm not sure.

But when she's not able to come up with a cognitive response or the proper response, she'll do her counting. It's almost like an anxiety-controlling kind of thing.

I asked what she was counting. She just kept on counting, so I decided not to pursue it. Instead I talked with her a little about her health. Right at that first meeting I intuitively and immediately felt that I wanted to work with her. I asked her if she had any visitors. No, she didn't, but she wanted to go home. "My husband might take me home." She talks about her husband a lot, and that's important in working with her. I have a feeling that some part of her knows that he has died. That's a problem that maybe we can talk about later. We had what I would call a small conversation. Her replies were brief but appropriate. I asked if she'd like me to come back; she said she would. I put it in terms of visiting once in a while; I didn't want to promise anything beyond that, such as an everyday basis, until I knew for sure. I thought that I could at least visit her on my lunch hour. That's how much I wanted to work with her.

I went then to the nurse and told her I had just been talking with Helen C. "*Talking* with her?" she said. "Yes, and she told me that she doesn't have any visitors and I asked her if she'd like to have some once in a while, and she said 'Yes.' " The nurse replied, "Well, she *doesn't* talk!" Indeed, when I read her charts later I found that one of the psychologists had interviewed her and reported not getting any response. So this is a beautiful kind of happening that we have here.

The nurse immediately went over and bombarded Helen with questions. "So—you want visitors! Why didn't you let us know you want visitors?" That sort of thing, almost accusative. Helen just looked at her. Finally, Helen said, "Well, yes. But not too many." And I thought the nurse was going to flip or flop! So I spoke with Ted Barber and Cheryl Wilson—both staff members of the Special Projects Division—and asked if I could work with her. It was brought up in the patient care meeting that she did respond to me, and my working with her became official.

Since she's been at Cushing there has been a big sign: "Feed Patient." She always has to be fed. Her legs are really contracted, but her arms seem less rigid; she has some range of motion with them. I spoke to the Physical Therapy department about that, and she is getting some help with range of motion. Other than that, Helen simply lies in that bed day after day. She doesn't get up. She has a decubitus on her upper buttock area, and the staff is concerned about skin care if she's sitting up for any prolonged period of time. I thought I would work rather intensely with Helen and get that decubitus healed. I've already started working toward that goal by telling her how much healthier she's becoming day by day, that sort of thing.

I did go back to Helen about three times a week for the last few weeks. She has become more and more cognitively responsive, more and more lucid in conversations with me. There is even a wit about her, really, a wit! Much more presence of mind.

My feeling was that Helen would need a lot of attention, would need to be visited almost on a daily basis, and not just for a ten-minute visit, but a real sitting-down with her for maybe half an hour at a time. I wasn't always able to do that. I have been able to see her only about three times a week instead of every day, and that bothers me. I have made it a point to make these visits as high in quality as I can. I take the time to really sit and talk with her. Ted (Barber) came down once, and she talked with him, too.

Something interesting is happening now. She will keep a moment of silence and then start the conversation going again herself. Usually I have been the one to start things. Yet the conversation she starts is not always factually appropriate, even though she speaks in a sensible way. When Helen converses with me, the nurses surround us at a little distance, watching and listening. She does not respond as fully to the nurses, but she now does exchange a few words with them. Physical Therapy has noticed this kind of change in her as well.

I noticed that she was eating more than usual, and in the course of conversation I started thinking more about what could be done to get her out of this bed situation. I had been talking with her about how springtime was coming, and what would be going on in the garden. The nurses will let me use one of those special chairs to bring her out to the garden, and she's looking forward to that. I have been trying to give her something to look forward to, not just the visits, but a kind of aiming toward whatever she has the potential for.

With this kind of thought in mind I wondered if maybe she could feed herself just a little bit. I had been working with another patient whom they thought could never feed herself. It really took a lot, but it worked; she was able to end up feeding herself. I thought maybe this could happen with Helen. She has not fed herself since she has been here, which is about six months.

I asked her if she could move her hands. She looked at her hands and then looked away. I touched her hand. Her arm and hand were very rigid. So I spent about five minutes holding and relaxing her hand, and when I thought that her hand was relaxed and comfortable —

Did she relax?

Yes, she did. I said, "Now, you can relax your muscles, just like you always did." I asked her to imagine doing something that she's always done so that she can relax and feel control of her hands. "For example, why don't you imagine you're playing the piano?" You know what she did? Helen's hands moved a little bit, and she said to me, "I used to play the piano. I have a piano at home. I *do* play the piano." She talked more about the piano and while she was doing this she became more alive, even excited.

Had you known that she played the piano?

No, it's not even on her record.

Why did you say that, then?

I don't know why. I just did. And when she responded, I heard all kinds of music in my head. I asked her, "Do you like classical music?" There was no response. I said then, "Standard music?" Still not much of a response, just sort of looking at me. Then I realized that maybe she didn't understand what I meant, and I said, "How about something like . . . 'Moonlight Bay'?" "Yes," Helen said, "I know that one." I told her that it was wonderful she had this music in her. "Once you play the piano it's in your blood. It's just in your blood, as your blood rushes through your being. If I brought you to a piano it would just come back to you. And if it doesn't come back right away, that's all right; I'll play it for you though I don't play well." Helen said she would like that and was quite excited. I was really beside myself! She was so excited about music and the piano, and she had almost forgotten about the feeding situation. I excused myself from Helen and spoke with the head nurse about what had happened. She immediately looked up her records. There was nothing about playing the piano or musical interests, just knitting and housewife-type things. The nurse became excited, too. "I have to tell you, Beverly, you get more of a response from her than anybody does. We're really happy about this, and you're welcome here any-time." The nurse went back with me and saw how Helen responded. She told me she'd be very happy if I would try to work with Helen on self-feeding, although she thought it would be an extremely diffi-cult thing to do.

Usually they gave Helen pureed food. But the nurse said, "No pureed food today; let's give her something solid." This turned out to be lasagna. I asked her if she liked raisin bread. I buttered a piece for her and broke it up. I thought it would help if I described the food to her because she's almost blind on things up close. It took some work, but after about five minutes she took that piece of bread in her hands and lifted it to her mouth.

Was this the first time she had fed herself in the hospital, as far as anybody knows?

That's right, and all the nurses came running! They were all ex-cited. I think the excitement might have upset her a little, so they left me alone with her. I told her that what she had done was won-derful. It was a great difficulty for her, and I was sensitive to that and praised her. I told her I was proud of this progress. She protected herself by saying, "Well, not too much, too fast."

Have you ever told her that you were going to heal or make her better?

I told her that I would help her, and that some people saw me as sort of a healer. That's how I was approaching it.

I fed her the rest of her meal because I had promised her that I was only going to have her do just a little bit, which was all that she wanted. I told her I'd be back. The nurse was so excited that she asked me if I'd be willing to do this two days a week "because this is wonderful. We just can't believe this." I said, "Surely." I said I would come back the following day, which was yesterday.

When I went back to see her yesterday, she was crying. Just lying there, crying softly. I wondered if maybe I had pushed her too much or something. I took down her bedside railing and put my arms around her. I told her I cared very much for her—I loved her. I let her know that I would work very slowly with her. I'd like to help her with a lot of things, not just learning how to eat again. We would find the right tempo together. As I was talking like this, she reached over and just rubbed and patted my hand. She had stopped crying but was still sad. I talked about how we all have sad days and happy days.

But Helen still played on my mind. Then something happened when I had my meeting with Bob Johnson, another member of the SPD staff. Lisa, Patty, and Andrea were there, too. He did a yoga meditation that included a breathing exercise. He was telling us to touch our foreheads, to get in touch with the "I am" of ourselves, and I was really going with this. Just then an incredible thing happened to me. I thought I saw—literally saw—a vivid white light. I can't begin to describe it. Within the white light there were fiery colors. And there in front of me—face to face—was an image that I've experienced throughout my years. I haven't told you much about this. It was a Christ-like image of someone. Very Christ-like, looking at me. I sort of gasped; they told me later I said, "Oh!" While Bob was leading us further into the meditation, this vision was saying, "Come with me." I was having a conflict, trying to listen to Bob at the same time. It was almost like a hypnotic trance. I went with the vision, and I just left. I had a sort of amnesia and the next thing I remember, Bob was suggesting that we see our patients while we are meditating. This is something he often does. We think of this as *a kind of absent being-with* the patient. Immediately, I was looking right into Helen C.'s eyes and seeing her, just looking at her, and feeling so much love for her. As this happened to me, the Christ image went right around me and behind me. It was as if I were looking out of more than one pair of eyes, do you know what I mean? I felt an incredibly beautiful experience going through me.

The first time?

Yes, yes it was. That experience I described, which I guess you could consider mystical, I do, stayed with me throughout the evening. I felt myself thinking about Helen and questioning in my mind why she was the one who became visible to me instead of any of the twelve other people I've been working with. I felt it was probably because she was crying. She was tugging at my heart. I continued to think a lot of her that evening and sent her my whatever-it-is: I prayed for her, I guess.

When I went to see Helen the first time after this incident, I wondered if I had pushed her too much, getting her to eat the bread herself, and then having found her crying the next day. I felt she was having a conflict. There's a part of her that wanted to come out of her disability and be more independent again, and there's a part of her that was quite comfortable with the way she was. This is my speculation, anyhow. As it turned out, the next time she was willing to do more. I didn't have to go through the preliminary phase of taking her hand and putting it on the bread. As soon as I told her, "We have wheat bread today," she asked, "Where did it come from?" I told her it came from the kitchen. Then she looked across to the other bed and said something about the pillows. The other bed not only had two pillows but some stuffed animals—and at the foot of the bed there was a big teddy bear. Helen first mentioned the pillows. I asked, "Can you see those pillows?" She said, "Oh, yes, I see them, and I can see you." She said something about "that big object at the end of the bed." I told her what it was and she agreed: "That's right; it's a teddy bear."

The nurse came over a little later and I told her that Helen had noticed objects on the other bed. "Oh, she didn't see those things!" the nurse replied, and went on about her eye condition. "Yes, she did!" I insisted. So the nurse went over to the other bed, held up the teddy bear, and took it for a walk. "Do you see what this is, Helen?" "No, no!" Helen said, "It belongs over there! Leave the teddy bear over there; that's where it belongs!" It was obvious that she had more vision than people thought. During that session, Helen also started drinking juice by herself. That was a first. Since she has been here, she has never taken a drink by herself, or held her food and eaten by herself. Now she does these things. Helen also started to use her spoon. She has some extra difficulty because her vision for nearby objects is not too good. She had to hunt around a little to locate the bowl. But once she found the bowl, she tried getting food on the spoon and bringing it to her mouth. I worked with her very closely while she was trying to feed herself, making it as easy as I could without taking the action away from her.

As this was happening, the aides surrounded me, watching. They wanted to know what I was doing. Helen's progress seemed miraculous to them. A couple of times I turned to them and said something, hoping that Helen didn't hear me, because I do not like to talk about a person as though they are not there. I said to the aides, "You really have to be intuitive. Watch for the right moment, the right occasion, and use it." At that moment she was having difficulty, so I just gently placed the food on the spoon and gave the spoon to her so she could continue. She would try these actions over and over, a trial-

and-error procedure. I was extraordinarily patient with her because that is what was needed. Finally, she mastered it. She was able to feed herself. It was quite wonderful!

Something else. Not only was she noticing more and more things around her, but after she would eat a certain amount of food, Helen would take her bib and dab at her mouth. Very delicately, very lady-like, she'd take the bib as if it were a napkin. Helen was not just putting food into her mouth, even though that was a big achievement in itself. She was now enjoying a meal and using all the appropriate behaviors.

I often spoke to her throughout the meal. I'd say things like, "I'm so proud of you and I'm so happy to see you doing this." She would look right back at me and give me this little smile as if she were not only proud herself but also proud that I was proud. After the meal I would sit at the edge of her bed and just sort of pat her hand. We would sit there for about ten minutes in silence. Once in a while one or the other of us would smile.

The last time I was with her I had a young woman with me, Judy Doran. I was helping her get acquainted with the hospital because she was interested in working here in somewhat the way that I do. Judy interested Helen. The nurses say that Helen is now a little more responsive to them, but not the way she is with me. She did feed herself breakfast this morning but didn't try to feed herself at noon. She's being a little selective. I feel that within a month or two, even sooner, she'll be responding well to others.

I have been seeing Helen every day, and what I have just reported brings us right up to today.

Judy Doran's Report[4]

I want to bring up Helen C. today because I think this is a good case of transition from one therapy to another. Helen has made such progress in the past few months that the staff is in on it, too. They have started noticing how much she has improved and, in turn, they are paying more attention to her needs. Before Beverly started working with her, Helen was a very isolated patient who stayed in bed all day and didn't talk, except for some random counting. You know the rest from Beverly's account.

4. This report was made six months after Beverly's report.

I met Helen when I first went around the wards with Beverly. Helen responded to me, too. I told her what I was doing and that I was hoping to get a job here. Helen said, "Well, I hope you do get a job here. It's a very demanding type of work." It was unusual for Helen to be so responsive and to answer in such long sentences.

The first time I started working with Helen I found her curled up in a fetal position. She speaks very, very softly. When you talk to her you have to get your ear right down to her mouth. This is the only way you can hear what she is saying. She would answer questions in a very few words, but she would answer. The next time, I tried to see if she would eat for me, too, as she had been for Beverly. She did take a few bites for herself, but that was about all she would do. She was having trouble seeing. Helen could make out shapes, but I think she couldn't see well enough to pick up the spoon all the time.

We asked for an eye consult. The attendants then found out that she did have a pair of post-surgical glasses in her drawer that had never been placed on her. But once Helen had the eye consult, the head nurse told the attendants to put the glasses on her every morning. They have been doing this, and it really does help Helen. She is a lot more aware now.

The technique I use is very gentle, very supportive, with a lot of positive suggestions to help her realize that she still can do things for herself.

Examples?

When Helen talks to me it is often in terms of, "I can't see, I can't walk, I can't do this, I can't hear!" I tell her, "Well, Helen, you can hear me. You're communicating very well right now!" I tell her that sometimes it is really distracting on the ward, what with radios playing, patients crying. I ask her to tell me how many fingers I am holding up, and see how well she can see. Helen is able to do little tasks and answer questions like this, and this helps her realize that she still has abilities. I encourage her and praise her successes. I always greet her with a gentle touch. Sometimes I hold her hand, sometimes just sit quietly, letting her know that somebody is with her.

I've been seeing Helen daily. I see her two times a week for feeding, and the other three days I visit with her and talk. About a month after I started working with Helen she was given an adjustable reclining chair. Before this, she had been in bed all the time. The nurses would turn her, but she would always be in bed. When she was moved to the chair, Helen became much more alert. We all noticed a difference. The nurses started commenting to me about her progress, and notes of this kind also started appearing on her chart. They would document that she is eating, she responds, she is communicative—things that were never documented before. A few weeks later I put a note in the chart myself to document that fact that she had now eating an entire meal by herself on some days. One day she was doing so well that she even refused my help. She was eating jello and having a hard time with it on the spoon. "Do you want some help?" She said, "No, no!" and pushed my hand away—and did it all herself. I also noted that she is alert and communicative when spoken to, although, by nature, is probably a quiet woman. She does not initiate conversation but likes visitors. She speaks frequently about wanting to see her mother. She's disoriented to present time and place.

Does she ever give indications that she knows her mother is dead? In other words, does she always express the desire to see her mother, or does she have two kinds of reality: that her mother is dead, and that she wants to see her anyhow?

This is really interesting. Helen, I think, sometimes knows that her mother is dead and at other times she thinks her mother is at home and that she has to go home and see her. She seems to have a lot of guilt about her mother's death. Both Helen's mother and her own daughter died of pneumonia. Helen talks a lot about her mother being in the hospital; she just has to go and see her. Yet at one point I asked, "Where is your mother?" "She's in heaven," Helen replied. That day she was clearly aware that her mother was dead. The next day she was saying again, "I want to see my mother; *I have to see my mother.*" She was sounding very anxious. After she spoke so anxiously about having to see her mother, I asked Helen again: "Where is your mother?" And she told me, "She's in heaven, I hope, but maybe in hell." From conversations like this, I think she is really worried about what happened to her mother.

Have you explored Helen's feelings about her mother?

Yes. I have asked her about her mother and father when it comes up sometimes. Her relationship with her father was a little bit worse. She said one day that her father was coming home tomorrow. "Are you ready to see your father?" No, she said, she didn't want to see him at all. I think her feelings about her mother being in the hospital have something to do with Helen's own situation here at Cushing. Logically, Helen seems to recognize herself as an old woman in a hospital and at the same time she thinks that her mother is around. I think she thinks her daughter is at home, too. She spoke about her daughter once, saying she was nineteen years old and very sick. From what I read in the chart, the daughter did get very sick and die at home of pneumonia. I try to accept where Helen is because it changes from day to day.

The head nurse is very supportive of all that is going on. She has now referred other patients to me because of the progress she has seen Helen make. The attendants have also made remarks, saying that they are glad somebody is working with her because they realize Helen is a lonely human being with lots of feelings.

Lately, I'd say the past week or so, Helen has been getting angry at me when I try to push her too hard. I encourage her to eat, but if she doesn't feel like doing it right, then she yells at me. This is another good sign—she feels comfortable and can assert herself. She has a much stronger voice than I realized. The attendants will even turn around from their work and wonder who is yelling over there. Helen had always been so quiet, never a noise-maker. I think it's good that she feels comfortable and can express her anger right out. I think often patients must feel really afraid to show they are angry for fear of being rejected again, but I always let Helen know that it's okay to feel anger and that I'll still see her every day.

Has Beverly continued to see her?

Beverly was working with me for the first several weeks, but then she discontinued her visits. I visit her every day.

Does she ask for Beverly?

Once Beverly did go to see her on the ward and Helen did recognize her. She doesn't go on asking for her, though; I don't think she is that well oriented. She doesn't know me by name although she does know me when I come to see her.

What are your goals and objectives for Helen now?

I'd like to continue trying to reduce her feelings of withdrawal and isolation. I want to maximize her ability to feed herself and to do anything that she can do for herself.

CASE 8: GEORGE L.

by Beverly Ryder

George L. is a sixty-eight-year-old man who had five brothers and two sisters. The next of kin is a brother who hasn't been in contact with him since admission. It was said that George was a quiet boy who liked sports. He left school at sixteen and worked as a clerk in a bakery. When his tonsils were removed in 1931 it was found that he had a heart problem. Apparently this frightened him, and he worked very little after that time.

About four years later his mother noticed that George's thinking had become paranoid. He was treated at an outpatient clinic. The diagnosis was psychoneurosis with mental retardation. He was admitted to a state mental hospital at age thirty-four. George was generally healthy there but not interested in hospital activities. His symptoms were delusions, hallucinations, and overconcern with his health. Thirty years later he was transferred to Cushing, with a primary diagnosis of dementia praecox, simple type.

I began seeing George four and a half months ago. I had gotten to know him some before that, however, when he would speak to me on the ward or in the Captain's Chair (the recreation center). I had been seeing some other patients that were on his ward.

I had a referral to see him because of his manic behavior. Apparently this is a cycle he has gone through many times before. He was frightened, racing around the hospital, confused, difficult to manage, and voiding where he shouldn't.

When I first saw him, he was extremely upset. The nurses were considering jacketing him into a chair. I was able to persuade them not to do that, at least until after I had had a chance to work with him. I talked with George about calming down and helped him do so. I helped him acknowledge that he was afraid. He said that he was frightened because of his bronchial condition.

One outstanding quality about George was that he was obsessive about his religious belief. Sometimes he would talk continuously about God and saints and things like that. Rather than avoiding that subject, I went with it and told him we would talk together about religion since it meant so much to him. I told him that he was a good man. I made a big point of that: "You are certainly a good man, George." I also spoke of the love of God. He should let God's love calm him and help him with his fears. I would be there to help him, too.

There was an immediate rapport. He would look at me with absolute trust in his eyes. I felt strange being the object of so much trust. You could just see the trust. It got so that after a while he'd calm down immediately when I entered the room even if he had been very upset. I'd put my hand on his shoulder, and he'd immediately calm down. The nurse came to me a couple of weeks after I started working with George and asked, "What is it you do? Tell me, so I can do it, too!"

When I wasn't on the ward, they would page me if George was getting very agitated. I saw him twice a day for the first few weeks. He really was very frightened. I talked with him about his fears. I told him that everyone is afraid some times and how I used to be afraid. I told him I would help him with these fears. You could see his fright in the running away, the suddenly jumping up, and especially in his eyes. I recognized this fear as the fear of dying. The health problem was triggering it. I don't think he himself saw it as the fear of dying, but the fear was so strong with him I felt that it was not appropriate to approach that subject with him. I wanted to get to that someday, but not at this time.

Check me out: you felt that the fear he was expressing in his behavior and his manner was essentially the fear of his own death, but that he wasn't ready to acknowledge or be confronted with that?

Exactly.

And what made you think that death was behind his anxiety?

The religious preoccupation. He wanted so much to be good and to be assured a heaven. He made those kind of connections in his conversation. And he talked about *The Nun's Story*, a book that I had read when I was a young girl myself. I found a copy of it in large print in the library, and he read it. I was assured by the librarian that he did read it. As a matter of fact, she was concerned about getting the book back. He would discuss that story, and we would talk about nuns and health.

Although he is preoccupied with health, George is an avid smoker—worse than me! I did tell him that it would be helpful if he cut down on smoking, but mostly I worked on relaxing him. He was very responsive to positive suggestions. I incorporated his religious inclinations into the relaxation therapy. "George, I'm going to help you relax." I'd put my hand on his shoulder and he'd look at me very trustingly. "I want you to relax your whole body." Then I'd go through a relaxation exercise with him and explain it as we went along. I told him this would help his body become free for healing to take place—and that the love of God would help him relax. And he did become totally relaxed, almost like slipping into a trance state. He'd just sink right into the relaxation. I had asked him about things that he found pleasant, and I used these as the basis for relaxation images.

George was having particular trouble in going to sleep. When he would get into the relaxed state and was listening to me, I'd say, "Now, George, you know how good you feel now, so relaxed and calm." He said, "Yes." "Now, tonight when you go to bed, imagine that you are at this summer resort. Think back to that time, to that good time. I want you to imagine that you are there at this resort, and you are going to have a wonderful sleep." Actually it was more a camping-out arrangement, but George referred to it as a summer resort so I went along with that. "You are going to wake up feeling refreshed and good, and you're going to sleep all night long." And he did! The nurses told me that he slept through the night, night after night. He told me that he had done what I suggested and had slept well. I also reinforced that God was helping him; and he should relax and let God continue to help him.

I never did get the chance to work on his death fear. That is still unresolved. However, he did get better and I saw him regularly for two months. Then I cut my visits from twice to once a day and then to about twice a week and, finally, to "on call." I worked closely with nursing. They said that it was remarkable how he was on this "high." That is how they referred to his state of mind. I saw it very differently. I saw George as a man who was in terror and needed a lot of company and reassurance. But whatever you call it, George did very well. He began going back to recreation therapy, was less of a problem, and was sleeping much better.

You've described how you worked with George. Could you say a little about what he looked like, and also be more specific about the ways he was behaving that might have led nursing to interpret him as being on a "high"?

He's tall, thin. His face looked tortured, but he was full of energy. This energy has a lot to do with George being seen as on a manic high. Lots of quick, jerking movements. His eyes would dart in terror. A kind of racing, a getting-up quickly to run away, as if running away from the situation. Trying to run from his fear—a haunted person. It's hard for me to talk about this because I'm feeling so much of what he must have been experiencing.

And this man is within the context of a geriatric hospital where behavior is generally slow-moving and without a superabundance of energy. A person with unpredictable sudden movement who has the energy to move around and whose thoughts are not well known to other people—and with a psychiatric diagnosis to establish his reputation—couldn't he be frightening to other people?

Yes. The patients were afraid of him. And what was interesting was that George was more afraid of *them*. He talked to me about being afraid of other patients. I said that this was understandable and reassured him that nothing bad was going to happen to him.

What was he afraid of in other patients—that he would be hurt physically?

Yes. At the time there were three other patients on the ward who were fairly new and who were disturbing other people. There was talk that they had pushed or hit some people, so there was some fear around, whether they had actually done anything or not.

George made it to the point where he was able to maintain this calmness without my being there. I would tell him to imagine that I was there if he felt frightened. I was considering making a tape for him for the weekend, but then he got better so it didn't seem necessary. It might be necessary for me to start working with him again some time, and a tape[5] might be useful.

Something else was happening at that time. Don M. (another patient) was very sick. George was very concerned about Don. "Is Don all right? He's not here!" I offered taking George to see him on the ICU. He was very hesitant. He wanted to see him, but also seemed frightened about it. I thought maybe he was afraid that Don was going to die, and he would be facing a death situation. It might

---

5. The holistic therapists sometimes record a program of suggestions and images particularly suited for the client, who then can listen to the tape whenever desired.

be too much for him. Finally, one day I knew Don was doing better, and George said again, "Let's go see Don." He had said this before, but then would decide to put it off. This time I did take him to the ICU. Just as we were getting near—I was holding his hand—George started pulling at me, "I want to go back! I want to go back!" I asked him what the matter was. "It's all right, George, Don's doing fine. He'd love to see you." George was shaking, he was so scared. After I reassured him, he stopped shaking and just stood still for a moment. Finally he did walk into the ward. Maybe I should have not done that. Maybe I should have let him walk away from it, but I did kind of persuade him to go in. George *stood* there. Poor George looked at Don. You could see exactly what it was: he was terrified. He couldn't get out of there fast enough. But he wanted to reach out his hand and touch Don.

Did he?

Yes, he did. He patted Don, and he said, "I'll be seeing you." Then out the door he went! I practically had to run after him. When we were walking down the corridor together, George said, "Well I saw Don. Don's all right. He's going to be all right." I said, "Yes, he is, George, he's going to be fine—and you're going to be fine, too."

I also explained to George about his immune system working better. This happened one day when he had a fever. "I have a fever. I might have pneumonia," he said. "Well, George," I said, "a fever is your immunity system going to work. It's fighting off all the bacteria that don't belong in your body. So that's good, isn't it?" George appreciated this explanation. Apparently nobody had ever explained the value of a fever to him. He had seen fever only as a bad thing.

George did get a lot better, and I didn't work with him for a while. Then the ward called me again. George was going into his cycle. They wanted me to get to him right away so he wouldn't get as bad as before. I went in and just put my hand on his shoulder and said, "Hi, George," and he relaxed immediately. I told him I was going to be seeing him again. "Good," he said, and then he was fine. I continued seeing him for about a month. It was not as intricate as before, more in the way of reinforcing what he had accomplished the first time around. He was always happy to see me, and he'd hold out his hand with the look of absolute trust.

I think with George it helped that I had beliefs not too different from his. He said, "You believe, too, I see you believe." Yet, I was sneaky, too. I presented the God he believed in as a God of love, peace, and energy.

When I see George on the ward now he walks right over and reaches over to shake my hand; then we sit down and talk together a while. He is in good shape, well controlled. The only thing else he seems to need to be happy is cigarettes. He is always looking for cigarettes.

God, cigarettes, positive reinforcement, and some love! I think it has to be said that you obviously like George: you like most of the people you have worked with.

I do, I do. I love them.

CASE 9: MARY P.

by Lisa B. Hathaway

Mary P. was born in England and, at age eighty-nine, had outlived her two brothers and one sister. Twice married and twice widowed, she had three children (two sons and a daughter) from her first marriage, all of whom now live in Massachusetts. After the death of her second husband, she lived alone until 1971 when she moved in with her son.

Although suffering several bouts of pneumonia, she had been basically healthy all her life. Soon after she turned eighty, however, Mrs. P. took several falls at home. After being admitted to a local hosptial, she was found to have Parkinson's disease. She could no longer be left alone at home, so arrangements were made for her admission to Cushing Hospital. At the time the therapeutic contacts began, she had been at Cushing for more than seven years. Ward notes included the status summary: "Given a certain amount of encouragement, she will answer questions. She is alert, independent, determined, and oriented, although she becomes nervous under stress and has some memory loss. She enjoys quiet and watching television." Mrs. P.'s condition had deteriorated from this level when Lisa Hathaway first met her.

Mary P. was sound asleep when I walked onto the ICU. I had never met her before and knew nothing of her. I had been working in the side rooms and, for some reason, instead of going into the office to write up a note on another patient, I just found myself walking to her bed and standing in front of her while she was sound asleep. I just felt naturally drawn to her all of a sudden. I thought afterward: "What am I doing here?"

And so, I just started working with her! I stroked her forehead, patted her hand. I felt compelled to flow curative fluids into her, give love to her, create a harmony. I felt in-balanced, even though she was sleeping beautifully. I felt there were a lot of things ruffled up inside her, even though she did not wake up while I was with her. After I left her I went immediately to the nurses' station and said I wanted a consult to work with this woman. They asked me the reason. I said, "I'm not sure yet." This kind of frustrated them.

It turned out that she had death wishes and she just decided very clearly that she was ready to die. She refused all fluids and all food and became dehydrated. They had to put in clysis to her.

She was an Englishwoman and a terrific actor. A couple of times she would play dead. Then, a little while later, she'd open her eyes to see if anybody was there, and she'd just relax. Often I was there when she didn't know it, just watching her. She was such a delightful woman to work with, but I had a problem of deciding what I was working for. The staff would say, "I don't see any improvement. Sure, she's a lot more alert, but she's *not eating*." I said, "What's the point? Am I here for you to keep her physical body alive or am I here to give her what I can for her mental status, her personality, to give her what she needs? You can't even *see* what she needs right now."

Did you say that to the nurses?

Yes! I was furious because they kept saying she was not eating. I kept looking at them and thinking—well, what's the point, am I supposed to be a nurse, too, and shove food down her throat and say, "Here it's good for you!"? At the same time I would be ignoring what was really happening. The nurses were trying to take care of the effects. I saw my job as trying to take care of the causes. So I had to be really firm with them because they just seem to miss the point a lot of times when we are working with patients. They would be really rough with me, with their tone of voice, for example. I would come right back to them cool and calm, but I'd get the point across. Now let me tell you what happened when I was working with Mary P. I had to say something about what was going on with the nurses and myself first because that was a real part of the picture.

Her speech was incoherent and garbled. She talked more clearly in her sleep. It was still a mumble, but the words were there, soft words, and you could pick them up sometimes.

She talked clearer in her sleep than awake?

When she was awake she mumbled on and on how she wanted to die. The garbling and the mumbling were different. In the daytime it was more of an anxious kind of thing where one word would just trip over the other, and you couldn't make any sense of it whatsoever. But at night, every once in a while a sentence or a couple of sentences would come out, and they were softly spoken. Sometimes she'd just whisper them; sometimes she'd mumble them a little louder.

How did you know that she had death wishes?

That goes back to the time I asked for a consult to work with her but couldn't give a reason for it. I had no doubts in my mind that she needed me and that I could help her, but I didn't know anything beyond that. Well, I did have this psychic kind of feeling that something was ruffling inside her, but I didn't think this would make sense to the staff. When I made my request for the consult, they said, "Well, she does have death wishes!" And they decided to make that the basis for the consult: the death wishes along with her refusal to eat and drink and whatever.

It was really a pleasure working with Mary P. She respected where I was coming from and she never really wondered who I was. I told her my name, but I really never told her that I was there to do healings with her or to work on her death wishes. I was just there. She began to trust me. As our relationship formed, it was a nice, natural thing. One time I came in while she was sleeping and placed one hand on her forehead and the other on her hand. She must have felt me being there because she placed her hand on top of mine, and though she never opened her eyes, she patted me softly on my hand and continued to sleep. It got to the point that she knew my touch, and she knew that I was there. This was only a few days after I started working with her.

She kept talking in her sleep, and the words became clearer as I continued working with her. There was a significant change in her everyday life. Everybody noticed that she had become more alert. Before, they would have to use a strong stimulus to wake her up, something physical. I felt this was because she didn't *want* to come up. She had a fear that if she woke up and was responsive, then they would start putting food down her—and she wanted to act as death-like as she could so nobody would bother her.

How do you know that?

I know that because I know her and from when I was working with her, I just felt . . .

Come on, Lisa. Did you have some clues to work with? Did she ever say anything to you about this? How did you form these impressions?

I watched her with the staff and heard what the staff had to say about her. "She always does this. She always does that. She always garbles." But as I worked with her, everything became clearer, her speech and her reactions. She wasn't afraid. She was coming out of her shell. She wasn't afraid to do that after a while, do you know what I mean and . . . what was your question?

You said that she would go into a kind of psychological hiding so that she wouldn't get food shoved down her throat. That's a pretty strong statement, and it may be true, but I still can't see how you came to that conclusion.

All right. At mealtime, that's a good example. She knew when mealtimes were. She could hear the banging and clanging of dishes and whatever, waking everybody up. "Come on, let's eat!" is what the sounds would say, and sometimes the staff would say it in words. This is when she would curl up in a fetal position and put her hands under her neck so nobody could get her hands. Or she would cover her mouth, or she'd really just form more of a shell with her body. She did this at those particular times of the day rather than any other times, and it just seemed clear to me.

That's a good observation, and it makes your conclusion more understandable. How much of what you and the others do can be made clear to people not in the situations themselves? That's part of my purpose here, Lisa. There may be some important things in the situation that cannot be communicated easily, but I will continue to try to get out of you everything that can be communicated in this way. This is not intended to make you self-conscious about things while they are going on, but we have to reflect upon it, I think, and see what really took place.

I can tell you more about this. A few days after I started working with her, I could feel her shutting out the world, yet *reaching* at the same time. I know that you are going to have umpteen questions about that, but that's what happened, and I wrote a note about it at the time. She was pulling away in general, but when I was with her she was trying to reach—ah, this is so hard to explain! Sometimes when I was with her I could see her just closing up like a clam, opening and closing at her own will and being protective of her situation. She wanted to be in control and was afraid of losing that. But there were times, more and more, when she would share with me, when she didn't feel vulnerable. I'm surprised that she opened up to me as readily as she did. Within a few days after I started working with her, she became comfortable. She didn't feel I was there for any reason other than for what she wanted herself.

Let's see if we can take it a step further, not with umpteen questions, maybe just half an umpteen. Suppose that someone else were watching Mary when she was opening up her mind as compared to when she was closing up. What differences would this person observe, visible differences? Did it have something to do with her posture, the direction of her eye contact, or things of that nature? I know you won't let me put words in your mouth; you never do.

The first couple of weeks that I started working with her, she refused to open her eyes, though she did start to respond verbally to my touch and my voice. After I while I challenged her. I said, "You know, I was taught that when you spoke to somebody you opened your eyes." And I added, "Aren't you the least bit curious about what I look like?" Finally, one day—and I'll never forget this—she thought that she would be funny and she opened her eyes. She more than opened her eyes. She bulged them and said, "See, I opened my eyes when you talk to me!" She was a very humorous lady, really cunning. Later on she did open her eyes in a normal manner, and she wanted to know what was going on around her, which I thought was good.

You moved a step ahead. Let's move a step back, just to be sure of details. During the first few sessions you were talking to a woman who had her eyes closed. You said she refused to open her eyes. How do you know it was refusal? All you can say is that her eyes were, in fact, closed. "Refuses" implies motivation, purpose. As it turned out, you seemed to be right, as usual, because when you teased and worked on her she did open her eyes and commented so as to suggest that her eyes had been closed on purpose and were now opened on purpose. Not a physiological matter, but her own intentions. Check? Check.

I would always spend a lot of time with her, and I would always feel this flow of energy, a peaceful kind of energy going through to her. I felt a gray fog around her a lot of times, something that the energy would have to get through. She certainly knew what she wanted, but she couldn't see it clearly. I wanted to reinforce what she wanted for herself, and help some light get to her through that fog. I would talk to her about living and the different options we have, the positive and the negative. At times we'd go for a couple of days in a row just talking about dying.

Could you give some examples of your conversations?

I will. I made notes right after them. I want to give the gist of it first, though. I felt that she knew what she wanted but did not really know what she was getting into. This is what made the fog image. Can I give some light? Can I help make things clearer verbally and give her a warmth from me that would make her feel comfortable with what I was saying? Can I make her feel comfortable enough to open and listen and still pick and choose what she wanted? I wanted very much to have this bond with her. Sometimes when I walked away I felt as if I had been preaching to her in a subtle way. But then I thought about it afterwards, and it always seemed to fulfill a need that she had. It would pop up in another question or whatever. So I definitely went on my own guidance. I never knew what I was going to say when I got in there.

We went for a period of time with no mention of death. We were just talking about life and living. She kind of maneuvered back to life for a little bit, and I thought that that was very important; but I wanted to help her in *either* situation. I wanted to help her when she wanted to live, but I didn't feel a great need to talk her into living on and on. I would be there if she wanted to die, and be there just as strongly. I wanted to be her support system either way. I was drawn to her.

She had lost fifteen and a half pounds since August and it was then October and she weighed only eighty-five pounds. She was a tall, skinny, still very delicate Englishwoman. She woke up while I was with her. She wasn't startled or anything. The light was on, and she gazed at me. I told her who it was with her, and that I wanted to stay if it was okay. She gave me the okay and fell back to sleep. I just wanted her to know that she still had the control as to whether I was there or not. Even though I knew she wanted me there, I thought it was important to give her that option. There isn't a heck of a lot you can give them at this point, anyhow.

Another time she woke as I was about to leave, and she stared at me. I told her to have beautiful dreams and that I would be back.

She seemed to like that. She was still at that time refusing food and fluids and was very tearful whenever they tried to give her anything. I felt so bad for her. But if they didn't give her nourishment by mouth, they would have to give her the clysis. No matter what was happening, she didn't like any of it.

Exactly why was she refusing food?

She was just ready to die. She thought that this was the quickest way. She just wanted to do it in a natural way, refuse all input and just let her body go.

And you are going to tell me how you know that—

I don't know how I know that! That's what I felt she was doing. She told me in a most positive way, not in an anxious way, but very softly and clearly. She'd look at me and say, "I want to die. I have had a full life, happy; I've done so many things. Now I'm ready to do something else."

She told you that?

Yes.

That's not your interpretation, but what she actually said?

That's what she told me. Usually I interpret things before, and then later on I find it was true. A lot of time I will sit with patients and say what I think they are thinking. Later on they'll say how uncanny it is that I know what they are thinking about. So I always go with that. I always talk to them. Really, it's like I am talking to myself out loud, but I know they are listening. I say, "Well, I have this feeling that you might be feeling this way at this moment and maybe tomorrow you'll feel that way." And I just go back and forth, kind of play with it a little bit. I give them some play, too. I don't want to come in with this Big Serious Conversation every day. That's no fun. You can't be too heavy all the time.

I told her that recently I had been there for many nights, stroking her forehead to make her comfortable while she was sleeping. She said that she liked it. I asked her if she would like me to return. She opened her eyes again, looked at me, and said, "Yes." First I did a healing on her. Then I gently touched her and said a few words. I started to ask her questions. We would kid along, for example, about whether or not she was going to open her eyes today. My questions were to find out what was in her mind just then. Some of the questions were good, some were dumb. She would respond in different ways to the good questions and the dumb ones. "That was a silly thing to say!" "Yes, I just wanted to make sure you were listening!" Once I said to her, "You know something, Mary, I think you're cutting yourself short." This is when I walked away and felt like I was preaching—something that I didn't want to be doing. But these words seemed to fit at the moment. Before I walked away I said more to her along the same line: "You have something special that not all the patients here have, Mary, and that's a mind. A mind is a powerful thing—the wonders that can be pursued with it! Amazing! You can dream, you can hope, you can imagine. Without these things, dreams, hopes, imaginings, one has nothing. I would really like you to re-evaluate your assets. There comes a time when your physical body is a real drag. This comes to everybody. But if you have your mind, why, you can change the boredom of it all." She heard me, and then she fell asleep. I wrote these words down after my little sermon, and I know I said similar things in other ways at other times. I just wish I didn't write it down at all. It doesn't seem to be me. It seems to destroy the beauty of the whole thing. You try to be concise and remember everything that you said.

Are you sorry that you said what you did?

No, I'm not sorry that I said it. But when I wrote it down afterwards it just didn't seem right because I couldn't get the beauty of it down in the words that I used; it is not the same thing at all on paper. That really frustrated me, made me angry.

Mary's attitude, though, was not depressing. It was rather clear and simple: she wanted to die. I could feel the fog lifting. I could feel her clarity increasing. There was a sureness before that she wanted to die, and she still wanted to die, but everything is so much clearer and lighter around her. This is something I felt psychically with her. Nursing agreed that there was a change in the way she said things, and that her eyes were much more open, talking a lot more. But these changes didn't impress nursing very much. "She won't eat! She still won't eat! So there really wasn't any progress at all!"

One afternoon she played dead. It was time for her medication, and she played dead. The nurse mimicked her in the office. She showed me how Mary had her hands all folded and held her breath— and just let it out a little when she thought that the nurse had left, and opened her eyes then, too. The nurse just gave her a little smile and walked away. I don't know if she ever got her medication that time or not.

She *is* a terrific actor. Whenever she has a temperature taken, she screams bloody murder. The next moment she's humorous and in control. The improvement in attitude I can see is that she still wants to die but doesn't totally shut herself off from the world. She's a lovely lady and a joy to work with.

The next day there was no talk of death. I reminded her about the birds singing in the trees outside her window at home. I talked about her home and its atmosphere even though I didn't know anything about this woman. I just said that you seem like the type of woman who would be sitting by a window and have the bird feeder there and the birds in the trees. You'd be up at the crack of dawn to be out there with the birds. I went through this whole thing, and this beautiful smile came across her face when I talked about it. She held that smile for the longest time, as though many good memories were coming back to her. After a while she'd say, "Go on!"

By this time she would open her eyes when she spoke to me almost every time, though it was hard to hear some of what she was saying. I explained to her why she had the needles in her legs and how she could prevent the clysis by drinking some fluids. At this point her attitude was positive and she spoke about death very freely, with no reservations. She'd still like to die, but on some days it was not Number One on her list. She gave me a kiss on the cheek when I left. She also hugged my arm, pulling both my hands against her cheek. This lasted for ten minutes or so. She just wanted me to keep my warm hands against her.

This was a pivotal point but also a time of confusion. The nurses were saying one thing—she's not eating, no progress—and I was seeing such beauty. Usually when I work with a patient I know exactly how I feel. Somehow with Mary, I felt confused at this point when I was working with her. I was very clear in what I was doing. But then I would turn around and nursing would say, "Well, you *could* try and feed her because we can't get her to do anything. She seems to be responding to you."

It got to the point where I started doing nursing. I started feeding her Sustagin (a high-nutrition substitute that is easy to digest), and that really wrecked our relationship. I wish I had never done it. It went on for about a week. They would say, "Could you get some-

thing into her because we really don't want to give her a clysis."
I really got caught up in a whole role that I didn't want any part
of. Mary resisted. I got the food down but just seemed to be losing
everything that I had won with her. I just was really hurt inside. One
time when I fed her it took me about fifty minutes to get about
240 cc into her, and that was equal to a whole meal. But then I told
nursing, "Okay, this is something that you can do. I don't want to
be a part of it. I don't want to make this woman sick (because she
was getting sicker with all this pressure on feeding). I want to help
her. I want to re-establish my relationship with her." I seemed to be
losing, going backwards, and I was really upset with myself.

She had been coming back to life. They had her sitting up in a
chair for most of the day, where before she had been lying curled up
in a fetal position. She was still a bed-and-chair patient as long as I
kept giving her fluids patiently so she wouldn't need clysis. She had
to have 1,000 cc of fluids a day, which was a lot for her. I gave
her Sustagin; she vomited afterwards. I had a lot of guilt feelings; I
was almost in tears, thinking, if I didn't try to feed her, maybe she
wouldn't be so sick.

At this point I was really furious with the nurses, but they hadn't
done anything wrong. It was just that I had taken on something and
now I was sorry for it. I had to re-establish my relationship with
Mary if I could.

I told her: "This might come as a surprise to you, but you are very
much alive. Your body is functioning at a slower pace, but you certainly aren't dying. I would like you to think about continuing to
live. Think about it right now, Mary. You have succeeded in shutting
out the world by refusing to look or speak to your family and the
staff." I had a feeling that she needed to know that she was truly still
alive. There was so much confusion around her, and that fog was
back again. I said these things, too, because I wanted to find out
where she was at, to see if she would react.

She responded to that. She was very pensive, just thinking and
not giving out much. At this point the great fog that I saw around
her earlier was lifted, and I felt that she was not so confused any
more but weighted down instead. She didn't know which way to go
because I was her support and now it must have seemed that I had
dumped her, though not meaning to. I couldn't blame her for looking at it that way. In the meantime the staff was getting very inpa-

tient with her. "She won't eat, and she plays dead, and she does this and she does that, and we are really tired of the whole process!"

This was happening during the fourth week I was working with her. The nurses were wondering why I should bother coming in if I wasn't going to help feed Mary. A lot of negative things were happening at the time; everybody was fed up. When I was about to leave her that day, I said, "Take care in every sense of the word." It felt good that she opened her eyes and looked at me. It was kind of reuniting because I was hurt that I had destroyed the relationship, and now she was giving it another chance.

Did you ever tell her how you felt about forcing food upon her or anything of that nature?

I did. I told her that I was trying to rationalize it in my own mind, not really knowing why I was doing it except that I had been asked to feed her and was caught in a predicament. I said, "If you could just get this down, they won't have to put the needles in your legs." I felt that she was ready for it but not that fast. She was coming back to life, just coming back, and she probably felt, "Boy! You hit me with all this food as soon as I opened my eyes!"

Did you ever say to her, "I'm sorry I pressured you to take the food"?

Yes, I did. I was the only one she would take food for anyhow. She would take a couple of sips at a time, and I would constantly apologize for it. "I didn't mean to force these things on you; I will respect your wishes," and things like that. The next day was mostly nonverbal. A few times I spoke to her and she opened her eyes while she listened. Twice as I was soothing her forehead she'd just open her eyes to look at me again, without any words at all.

This was a Friday. She died early the next Saturday morning. That Friday we had a really beautiful session together. The nurses finally agreed to respect her wishes and not to force the intake. I sat one of the staff down and told her about my relationship—what had happened, how far we had gotten. I told her that I didn't feel that putting food into Mary was the way for me to be useful; I was ruining my own intentions with her. I didn't want any more part of it. The nurse replied then, "Well, we really should respect her wishes." I thought, "Well, it's about time." The nurses were flip with me this past week, about her condition worsening. They admitted her responses were good as far as being more verbal and opening her eyes, but the intake was still the big thing with them, the only thing, it seemed. I tried to make them understand that I wanted to respect Mary's options, not just to march in there and force my perspective or anybody else's on her. I considered my communications with her very precious and deeply want to be with her when and if she died. She asked me to be there also; Mary asked me.

You said the ward staff was "flip" with you in that last week. This isn't entirely clear.

I think they felt that I was doing a lot of nonsense with her—as if I were just holding her hand and not really accomplishing anything because the things that were happening were really subtle between her and me. Nurses who walked by every ten or fifteen minutes weren't really going to pick up anything that was going on. That's half the problem with our therapy. We are not moving legs and arms, and we are not doing a "project." We are working one on one. Even though I'd tell them about the subtle changes, they were out of context for them. They couldn't understand. "So what? She's not eating!" A one-track mind. You couldn't tell them about the other changes and get them to understand or really to listen. It got to the point that you didn't want to tell them because you knew it would be ridiculed, not appreciated.

But is "flip" the word that really fits their attitude?

It felt flip at the time. They were very firm with me. "I feel you're not getting anywhere with her." They didn't understand what I was doing with her. They were flip with me in that anything I would say would get a short and sharp reply. That whole week was filled with tension.

That Saturday morning Mary died, very early. I felt pleased for her sake. I wish I could have been with her, I guess more for my sake. I have so much respect for her attitude and her strength, what she had to go through to do what she did. She always knew what she wanted, and I thought it was my job to make sure that she felt secure with the idea of dying. She respected me. She never refused to listen to what I said about options on living and dying. I felt that I learned a tremendous amount. It was at that point—with Mary—that I decided I am here for the patients. I knew this before, but I never really verbalized it to myself and never realized the kind of situation you can get into where somebody wants one thing, somebody else wants another. This makes you wonder who you are there for. At that point I made a stand within myself that I am here for the patients. And that's that! Oh, I learned a lot.

You mentioned the family briefly. Is there anything relevant that you can add about them?

I never met the family. The staff said that the family was upset because she wouldn't open her eyes and she wouldn't talk to them. She'd just lie there, and the family would be in tears because they'd be so upset that she wouldn't communicate in any way.

You were not there when Mary died. Do you have anything more to add about her death?

When I came back Monday, they said that she had died early Saturday morning. I thought back to what I was doing at that time. I was up early Saturday. I was stacking wood, and I constantly thought of her, but I never really thought of her dying. Other patients I picked up the sense, I mean, the feeling that they were dying right then. This didn't happen with Mary. No rush came through me. I was thinking of her, but not of her dying.

CASE 10: ALFRED B.

by Lisa B. Hathaway

Alfred B. is a seventy-six-year-old man who was transferred from a
state mental hospital five years ago after being there about seven
years. He has a brother and a sister, both of whom are still alive.
Mr. B. left school after the seventh grade and worked as a machinist
until he was nearly sixty. He never married. He has been deaf since
adolescence and has had increasingly poor vision since he was about
forty. Cataract surgery was performed, but he has been blind for several years now. It is thought that he can hear words when they are
shouted, and is reported to be responsive at a simple conversational
level for short durations. There is memory deficit for the recent past,
and instances of delusional thinking have been reported. In addition
to Mr. B.'s blindness and deafness, the medical history lists left lin-
guinal hernia and chronic brain syndrome.

Alfred B. was given to me at a patient care meeting, and I was
given one week to do something with him. He had recently moved
to a different ward and had become a behavior problem. This deaf
and blind man had had a private room but was now in a ward area
because there was no private room in the new ward. That automatically caused a lot of problems. He had to get reoriented, which can
be difficult enough for a person who sees and hears. Nursing said
that he had become disoriented. He was abusive, especially at night.
He wouldn't take his meds because he was afraid of being poisoned.
He had very poor hygiene and constantly spit on the floor. The
nurses' notes say things like this: "Very agitated—tipping over
chairs—throwing ashtrays through table and broke it—all other
patients moved out of the solarium—agitated during transfer—bothered another patient who had to be moved to another cubicle for his
own safety. He also tried to pull this patient out of his bed. . . . Unco-
operative, urinating on the floor. Refused to take off clothing. . . .
Noisy, disturbing to other patients, asking for cigarettes, constantly
urinating on floor."

The first time I went down to see him, the nursing staff said they
wanted to warn me about three things: he goes to bed when and if

he wants; he never uses his urinal; he doesn't like to be touched. I was trying to go in with a positive attitude, and that is what hit me!

I watched Alfred while he was in his wheelchair. He's a very small man. He weighed no more than 100 pounds, certainly. And he was just filthy, with food all over him, all over his hair. He didn't have much hair, but what he had was a mess. He was smoking away. He did find the ashtray next to his chair, which I thought was a positive sign. He continued to blow his nose in through his hands. The poor guy had nothing going for him at this point.

"What do I do now?" I asked myself, not really knowing. I decided to yell into his partially good ear. I asked him if he wanted a back rub. "No, no, I'm broken. I'm broken at the knees, thighs, waist." He showed me all the places he was broken, "Here, here, and here." He also stuck his finger down his throat at the same time, and then blew his nose into his hands again.

I decided to give him a back rub anyhow. He said again that his back was broken, and I said, "I really want to do this." I started gently on his neck. He said, "No!" three times, and was really loud and cross. I think this was supposed to scare me away, but I just continued to do it, really gently, on his shoulders. Then I started a little bit lower. Within about three minutes, he put his head to his knees so I could do his whole back. After about fifteen minutes he said, "Okay, enough. I want to go to bed." So I put him to bed.

Yourself?

Yes. I wheeled him to his bed. Oh—while I was doing the back rub, I was also doing a healing on him at the same time. I was concentrating on visualizing the peace that I felt inside myself and transmitting it to him. I really felt a lot of strength and vitality, going through me to him. I felt a lot of things happening. I would call it a mystical experience or state. I forgot about the time and I forgot about where I was. The next thing I knew is when he said, "Okay, that's enough," and I brought him to his bed.

Had you told him your name at this point?

No, I just told him I wanted to give him a back rub.

He got up from the wheelchair and said, "I want the urinal." It turned out that he had never used the urinal before. "Let me find one." So I found one and gave it to him. He said, "All right, take the chair away." He got into bed and into something of a fetal position, still fully clothed. He pulled the covers up to his head and he was freezing. I just sat there and watched him. He thought I had left by this point. He was cold; he didn't have a blanket on his bed. I wondered what he was going to do. He got up in a moment and felt around for his dirty old sweater and put it on. I kept thinking he should have a blanket on his bed.

I went back the next night, after he was in bed, and told him I wanted to give him a back rub. It was a beautiful session. The next night, the staff was very surprised. It was the first day he hadn't fallen. I guess every day he had had some kind of a fall, so he was doing really well. I want to read the conversation we had the second night.

I told him I wanted to give him a back rub and he said, "Get out of here!" I said, "Alfred, it will help to soothe your back." "My back is broken," he said, "It broke six months ago. There's nothing you can do. I only get out of bed to have a cigarette or a meal because of my back. You're new here, aren't you?" And then he gave this hideous laugh. It seemed to be at my expense, that I didn't know what the heck I was doing.

I said, "Yes, I am new here, why?" "'Cause I thought so. The state hospitals hire you girls and boys to do all the dirty work for them. This is a murder house. They put needles in your hips and paralyze them. They were supposed to fix my eyes, but they never did. They don't want me to see what's going on. The doctor gives you poison pills. All the state hospitals are doing this, doing the same thing."

I replied, "Alfred, everyone needs someone. Thank you for warning me. But I'm not yet convinced about what you say. I have not seen these things." He said, "You better watch out, or you'll be on the list, too. You'll find out. The guy in the next bed was killed last Sunday and another one the Sunday before." That's when I reminded him that he was the one who was trying to get that same man out of the bed and that this man had not died but had been moved to another part of the ward. I continued rubbing his back after this conversation. How he liked it! Finally he said, "Okay, good night. Go away now." I said, "All right, I'll be here tomorrow night." And it became a real ritual. I felt I didn't need words with him.

Now, you weren't, in fact, new there, were you?

No, I had been there for about ten months. I didn't give him my name because I didn't think it really mattered. He just knew me by my touch. I come to him at night and he's really relaxed. I just tap him on the shoulder and give him a back rub, and I say, "Hi, Alfred," and he goes, "Hi." Every once in a while he wants to know what time it is. I would continue intensely with the healings because I had only one week to do something with this man and I really felt sorry for him.

I started with him on a Wednesday. On the following Saturday night they changed the medication. When the next patient care meeting came up—Wednesday—they said, "He's doing so much better, but the medication's been changed, and that must have been what is doing it." Meanwhile I already had good results. The nurse kept reporting to me a lot of good things that were happening to him. So I just said to myself, "I'm not going to worry about that" (the assumption that the changed medication accounted for his improvement).

You said you had a week to work with him. Would you clarify that?

The patient care meeting came up with the recommendation to try human contact therapy for a week. I don't know the details of it. I assumed that if I didn't show a lot of progress in a week that human contact therapy might be abandoned. But I did continue to work with him for two months. I saw a lot of changes happening. First he was sleeping in the fetal position. A few weeks later he was sleeping on his side. Toward the end, he was sleeping flat on his back. When I started working with him he would pull the covers up over his head and let his hair stick out. Later, he would just have the covers up to his waist. It was body language for trust. He let himself be more vulnerable, less protected, because he started trusting his environment more. This was a big improvement, I thought.

Some of the nurses started to approach Alfred with more determination as he improved. They had not approached him much before because he must have seemed like such a hopeless case and did his best to keep people off. One attendant decided to wash him up before she wheeled him to bed. She said, "C'mon, let's get washed up." He just started to laugh at her and said, "I haven't been washed up in five years and six months." "Well, you're going to get it tonight!" She really stood her ground. She brought him up to the sink and gave him the soap and water. He washed his whole body, did a beautiful job. Then she gave him a back rub—and he loved it!

I was encouraging the nurses to help him clean up before putting him to bed. Once he got into bed, Alfred was not going to cooperate. There happened to be a few attendants who had a routine going of just getting the patients to bed as quickly as they could. They especially didn't want to get close to Alfred. They were afraid of him. This created a situation in which he was getting practically no contact. After this one girl took the initiative it made things easier, and they had a ward meeting to discuss how to care for Alfred. It made an impression on the others when this one attendant told them how easy it had been, how much Alfred had done for himself, and how he loved the back rub.

For my regular visits I'd go up and tap him on the shoulder and give him back rubs. I'd always do the healings because I could really feel things happening—intuitively—and I didn't want that to stop. He was now feeling very secure, no more of that murder house stuff. I felt we had a good nonverbal relationship, and he'd say good night as I was leaving. I'd pat his shoulder when I left.

Finally there came a time when it felt right to stop for a while. I suggested to him that we stop it for a while. "You can continue doing as well as you're doing now. I hope you've changed your mind about a few things about this hospital. I'd like to see you from time to time, but I'll give you a break now. I hope you're not upset. You know I was bugging you every night! All right?" "All right," he said, "good night." So that worked out well.

Would you go back to the healing? Say it again, as clearly as you can put it into words: what is it that you were doing with this man that you thought of as healing?

Healing to me is when I visualize something that happens. I can visualize my thoughts and it doesn't matter if I verbalize them or not. I can make my thoughts and visualizations happen within somebody and in any form that I want it to be. There are nights when I'd go in and feel really sensational—very trusting and secure and loving. I would just send that whole energy, and not just through the hands. It doesn't happen through your hands—well, sometimes it does, but it's channeled through your whole body. You feel a rush. One rush after another. You can just feel it working. In working with Alfred it was like a circle: I felt it going to him and then I could feel it coming back. It was a really tight bond.

You felt it coming back?

Yes, very mutual. It's always mutual.

You never said, "I am healing you" or "I will heal you"?

No, because that wouldn't have fit. He experienced me first as a fresh kid, somebody new there who was trying to give him a back rub, and did he really want it? He's supposed to be deaf, yet after a while I got to talking to him in a low voice and he got to talking to me in a low voice. He could hear me beautifully. That was much better than the shouting back and forth, and it helped to relax the situation. What happened was that one day I finally got tired of the shouting and talked to him in a natural, low voice, and he responded.

I do want to read you the monthly note they made on the 3–11:30 shift which was written near the end of the time I was working with him.

> Eating a regular diet. Alfred has made outstanding progress for us behaviorally. He's more agreeable and cooperative and has become nearly self-sufficient in ADL.[6] He still verbalizes little, only such things as "I want to go to solarium, bed, bathroom. I want a cigarette or a light." Alfred is less paranoid and is more social with staff. He is perhaps beginning to lose his delusions and fear.

He is still not what you would call a model patient, but he is feeling better about himself and is much easier for the staff.

How would you feel at the end of a typical session with him?

I'd feel terrific. A healing is always mutual. You get back what you put out. I always felt very satisfied; I always felt good. And I always stood at his bed and as I left—or as he thought I left—I would stand and watch him. And you know, it got to be where he was sleeping on his back and he'd have a half-smile on his face.

During this whole process did you ever make objective goals, such as, "I am trying to accomplish this and this and this"?

6. ADL: Activities of Daily Life.

I wanted to create a bond with him in some way. If he could come to trust me, then he might learn to trust other people and the hospital, the world.

Now he's still getting the back rubs at his p.m. care. He's getting attention he never had before, not just the basics. This helps to keep it going. He could still use more contact. He is blind, and doesn't hear well, although better than what people thought. A person like this needs a lot of attention and contact. The ward staff *is* doing more of that now; they kid around with him while they're giving the back rubs, for example, and they'll say, "You won't believe what Alfred told me tonight." There is something going on that wasn't there before.

CASE 11: MARIA F.

by Judy Doran

Born in Italy seventy-five years ago, Maria F. was one of five children but came to the United States by herself at the age of eighteen. She lived with a cousin in Natick until she married. Maria continued to live in an Italian-speaking community, first with her husband and son, later, when widowed, with her son and his wife. Apparently she never spoke much English and speaks even less now.

According to the records, Maria was a healthy person all her life until just last year. The first problem was a fractured ankle which led to hospitalization. When she returned home, Maria did not seem to be quite the same person. Her family noticed that she was really confused. One day she started striking out and was unmanageable. The family couldn't cope with her in that condition. Maria was then admitted to a local hospital, and came to Cushing four months ago. The diagnosis at admission was senile dementia, severe chronic brain syndrome, along with diabetes.

I started working with Maria after she had been here about a month. She had started on Ward A but was transferred to the intensive care unit about a week later because she had stopped eating and drinking. She was dehydrated. It was on the ICU that I started working with her. The nurses described Maria as a total care patient. She refused to eat, they said, and never said a word. A feeding tube had been placed in her nose so that she would have some nutrition. The nurses added something else: Maria would sometimes wake up in the night or when she was sound asleep and look terrified, really scared.

The Maria I saw for the first time was a very thin woman with big, expressive brown eyes. Those eyes conveyed a lot of emotion. She had her hands tied down to the bed because she had been pulling at the tube in her nose. She was lying in bed with the look of terror in her eyes. Her mouth was full of sores because she hadn't been eating. It was very dry. Her tongue was caked with dried skin. She looked very tense.

She had been sleeping on and off during the day. I went in to see her and held her hand for a while and just explained who I was—that

I wanted to help her, that I would be coming to see her every day to help her get well again.

I really wasn't sure how much she understood or if anything was understood. She didn't say anything back. At this point I didn't know if she even understood English.

I kept going back to see her every day. On the second day, in the afternoon, she did recognize me. I held her hand and she gave me a squeeze and nodded. I knew then that she was aware. Maria still looked terrified. I tried to put myself in her position. She was in a hospital where no one spoke her language, and I didn't think she understood what was happening. The nurses go by and everyone is busy. Unfortunately, the other patients are sick, too. She was in a room all by herself, really kind of isolated, and her hands are still tied down to her side. She probably doesn't know what is happening to her or why, so I tried to explain. I told her first where she was. She was in a room of her own. It was the room right next to the bathroom. Every time the toilet flushed it would make a loud noise, almost vibrate the walls, and that was alarming to her. She would look even more scared when that happened. I explained to her that what she was hearing was just the toilet next door flushing. At this, Maria kind of nodded and even smiled a little, as if to say, "Oh, yeah, I know what's going on."

That's basically the approach I used on the first series of visits; I tried to orient her to where she was. I would also ask her questions, and she sometimes responded to my questions either by nodding or squeezing my hand. Once I asked her, "Are you scared?" and that's when she told me, "Yes, yes!"

She told you?

Not verbally, by gesture. There was such a lot of nonverbal communication.

She'd communicate by squeezing your hand and by nodding her head, and what else?

Her *eyes.* She would get so wide-eyed. Once I tried to leave and she started to cry—wail, really—like she's very scared. That's the only way I can describe it. So I just stayed with her. I would try and calm her down, relax her. She responded to that. I think it was the third day I saw her. This was the first time she actually said anything.

Maria smiled at one point and then she said, "I like you." Those were the first words I heard her say.

At times I think she had really bad dreams, crying in her sleep. The nurses' notes would say that she's very noisy at night.

She did respond. I think she needed to be told that *"it's okay"* and not to be afraid. She is not alone here; she is in a hospital. Sometimes she would say the word "America" over and over—"America!" "America!" with an Italian accent. I think she said it in a sarcastic kind of way, as if to say, "So *this* is America? This is what I came all the way from Italy for?"

Did she speak in Italian?

She's all Italian. She speaks at great length in Italian now, really fast.

So in a typical visit—which you are talking about now—Maria might be saying a lot of words in Italian. How did you respond?

I would try to tell her that I didn't understand Italian. I only speak English. I don't think she realizes that we don't all understand. This doesn't stop her from talking; she talks on and on. There are times when I think she does make a strong effort to communicate. She can say a few phrases in English. She will say, "Hello" and "good bye," for example. I'll ask her how she is, and she will respond in English. I'll ask her how she is feeling. "Oh, not bad" or "Oh, not good," and then all the rest is in Italian.

A couple of weeks later Maria was transferred out into the ward, and she was a lot more responsive out there, with all the stimulation she was getting from just being able to see everybody walking around. It gave her a better understanding, I think, of where she was and what the hospital was all about. It was when she was moved out into the ward that I noticed she had this little doll in her bed. I don't know who gave it to her, maybe the family. She talks to the doll as if if is real.

In Italian?

In Italian.

Which the doll understands?

The doll understands. The doll "talks" to her and she talks to the doll. She smiles at it and laughs at it and kisses it and comforts it.

I think the doll is therapeutic for her. She seems to convey a lot of her feelings to the doll. When Maria is scared she tries to comfort the "baby." And when she wants someone to play with, it's baby again.

After she had been out in the ward for a few weeks, Maria started to notice that the patients around her were very, very sick. They all had the feeding tubes. They never got out of bed. It was a very depressing atmosphere. I think this got to her. She became upset again. One day the other patients were having visitors, and Maria was saying something in Italian about families and dying. One of the attendants spoke Italian, and she told me that death was a big part of Maria's commentary that day. And it was this same day that she was telling everybody that her *doll* was dead—her doll was dead and she didn't want it in bed with her. After a few days, however, she took the doll back again.

Were you able to discuss this with her?

I tried, but I'm not always so sure that she understood. I was trying to tell her that everybody on the ward was sick, but that they were getting better. I hoped this might help her to get better, too. I just wanted to let her know that everything was all right. I spoke to her then in the Italian I did manage to pick up. I speak a little French, which helps some. She would say things like *morte* for death: *morti mama, morti papa.*

Everybody's dead.

Her mother's dead; her father's dead.

Did she give you any reason to believe she might be thinking about joining her parents, reuniting through death?

She is a religious woman. She has a lot of religious Mass cards. I've seen her pray, and we talk about prayer. She seems to be praying *with* her father and mother and *to* them. I get the impression that she feels all alone, and does want to be with her mother and father. It was at this point that I asked the nurses if they thought Maria would be transferred to a different ward. They didn't sound too optimistic about it. They'd say, "Well, if she starts feeding herself and drinking by herself, then she can leave. Until then she'll be here for a while." But then just a few days later they did decide to transfer her. She went back to Ward A. That's where she is now. She's in her own little room and feels so much happier. The word that she has been using most often lately is *Benedicte*. She was saying that over and over, almost chanting, in Italian, the name of the Father, the Son, and the Holy Spirit. Over and over again.

Sometimes Maria seems to be in her own world. She will be talking to her doll about dying and death. But at other times she is a lot more tuned into the ward scene. In those moods she enjoys stimulation. Maria loves the attendants. They come in and check up, and she'll laugh and joke with them.

Last week one of the nurses had a birthday. Maria started singing "Happy Birthday"—completely in English! She is really in touch with a lot of what is going on around her. She likes to mimic some of the attendants and nurses when they walk by without stopping to call on her. Maria is a very expressive mimic and gets her sense of humor across as clearly as can be. She'll be joking and laughing behind their backs. She also mimics other patients. She did this even back on the ICU when Doris G. (case 2) was shouting, "Help, help, let me out of here!" These shouts scared Maria at first, but her attitude changed when I told her that what she heard was another patient who was upset. Maria then repeated the shouts she had heard, but in a joking, mimicking way.

What was your original goal in working with Maria, and what do you see as your goal now?

Originally it was a problem of adjustment. I wanted to help her adjust to the hospital and to understand what everything was all about. She really didn't understand that she was in a hospital, that she was sick. Now she is a lot more oriented to the hospital routine and to what she is doing here. She is still having fears about dying. This is what I want to help her cope with. I'm not quite sure what the best approach is with her because of the communication problem. At night she still wakes up, as though from bad dreams. The chart always says she's noisy at night. Perhaps they should give her some medication, that's her problem.

How about if somebody gave her some happy sleep talk, positive suggestions about sleeping well, and having dreams that are pleasant? This would be a very simple approach, but it might work. Tuck her in for the night, spend a few minutes with her. . . . How many patients had you worked with before you started with Maria?

Maria was one of the very first patients, the second patient I got that was "just mine." I had been working with Beverly Ryder on cases together, but Maria was one of the first I had all by myself. I started working with her the second or third week I was here.

You haven't described much in the touching, healing line with Maria. Did you or didn't you?

At the beginning I used a lot of touch with Maria. I was holding her hands. Sometimes that's all I'd do, just sit and listen to her speak in Italian for a great length of time. I'd just hold her hand all the while and tell her that it's all right and she's getting better.

Is she seen by her family?

They come mostly at night or on weekends. I don't know how often. I've never met them.

Do they know that you are working with her?

Probably not. Usually I don't have much contact with the family.

How do you usually feel yourself after you have seen Maria, say, on your most recent visit?

I feel good. I feel that I have an effect on her. I feel that she's calmer. When I leave I tell her that I'll see her tomorrow, and she goes, "Oh, good! Come again!"—in English. When I get an English response from her I feel really good about it. I feel like I'm making some contribution, some progress.

CASE 12: DWIGHT M.

by Lisa B. Hathaway

This man was born in Canada in 1890, one of eight children. Six of his siblings died in infancy because of respiratory problems. Dwight M. moved to the United States at the age of fifteen, and worked thereafter as a caretaker.

His neurological condition became evident when he was fifty years of age. It began with numbness in his toes and weakness in both lower extremities. His gait became staggered and he had to use canes. Five years later he fell and had severe back pain as a result. Taken to a major hospital, he was found to be suffering either from multiple sclerosis or amyotrophic lateral sclerosis, the differential diagnosis not being firm at that point. Several months later he was confined to a wheelchair, and he could no longer work. Three years later the condition made itself evident in his upper extremities with a very marked weakness, which finally resulted in a flexor contractive and spastic paralysis of the upper right extremity. The same occurred to a lesser degree in the lower right extremity.

He was admitted to a hospital that was engaged in experimental work on neurological disorders. The diagnostic assessment raised a question of an obstructive lesion in the neck, and it is probable that a laminectomy was performed, but there was no change in his condition. Since that time, he lived at home with his wife, receiving assistance from a visiting nurse. When his wife died twenty-one years ago, Mr. C. lived in the community for another two years with friends helping to look after him. He was admitted to Cushing Hospital nineteen years ago with a diagnosis of amyotropic lateral sclerosis.

Dwight is one of the patients that I would do a *sneaky healing* with. A sneaky healing is when you're working with one patient, you tend to comfort the surrounding patients in some way also. You do what you can for the people you have included in your caseload, and then you try to see the others on the side so they won't get jealous and there won't be any hard feelings.

Dwight had such a positive attitude that all the staff was drawn to him, including me. He was all crippled up. He could move one hand, but he couldn't do anything with the rest of his limbs because they were so contracted. He had been bedridden for thirty-seven years and lived at Cushing for eighteen of those years. I worked with him for nine months and a day. When I worked with Dwight I tried to bring him a lot of light, love, and reinforcement and whatever I could because he did a lot for me, inside, spiritually, just looking at him with all his physical limitations and all his suffering. He never had a bed sore, though, which is incredible.

After he died, I wrote this note:

8:10 p.m. Dwight died. The only thing that was keeping his body alive was his attitude. I'm trying very hard to find the right words to describe our relationship. He was one of the many patients I would do a sneaky healing on. A month or so ago, he looked at me with his very special smile and said, "May I ask you something?" He hesitated a little, almost afraid to ask. Then he said, "Do you love me?" I said, "Yes." The tears rolled from his eyes, he was so touched.

Everyone, including staff, would go to Dwight to be cheered up. I'd always bring him a kiss and a warm welcome. He was so delighted that I'd never hesitate to give him a kiss. He always thought, why would I want to touch him? He said to me many times that if he were younger and I were older, perhaps we could have a chance together. He asked me to marry him, even though he knew that it wouldn't be possible. He wanted the chance to propose to me. He told me of the girl friend he had planned to marry and how she died before they had a chance. It ended up that he married *her* girl friend.

He felt proud of his home, which he described in every detail, especially the piazza, which was his favorite spot. He would tell me how I'd love it there with him, music and all (he played the piano).

I got a chance to see him many times within these last few days before his death. Finally, three and a half hours before he died, I got to see him alone. I gave him the usual loving kisses and warm smile, and I even said some funnies that made him laugh, which wasn't easy for him. He was highly congested and didn't seem able to speak.

I took a moment to look into his beautiful eyes and said, "Dwight, are you dying?" He nodded his head and said, "Yes." He seemed relieved that I asked, even though I already knew what the answer was. It's just that nobody ever said the words to him. They'd say things like, "You're going to be okay" or "We'll see if you can make it through this one." But nobody ever said the word *dying* to him, so I felt it important that I say it.

I then said, "I have a favor to ask of you." He looked at me so surprised. I said, "Would you be my guardian angel?" He then smiled from ear to ear and laughed through his congestion as he nodded, "Of course." I told Dwight that I was counting on him, and I'd better be the first one on his list.

He tried to talk many times, but I encouraged him not to. He was far too weak. He then insisted. I put my ear next to his mouth and listened. I wasn't sure whether to look real close at him and listen, or with my ear to his mouth. It was very hard to hear. And then it all made sense. He repeated two lines again again: "You are beautiful" and "I love you." The tears came to my eyes. I was so overwhelmed. He squeezed my hand as I held his only moving limb against me. I held it under my neck and kind of against my cheek. I told him how very special he was. We both had tears in our eyes, and smiles on our faces while we continued to stare at each other.

By this time I had to leave and he knew it. I told him that I would return later that evening. It turned out that at the time he died, I was working with another patient on the other side of the hospital. I'm so glad I had the chance to say what he and I needed to share with each other. I felt that Dwight left me a tremendous gift of strength and inspiration. I felt really inspired by how he could have so much control from within.

About four months after Dwight died, I went to a spiritualist church and had a reading. The woman who did the reading said, "I don't expect you to know this name, but I just have to give it to you." And she said, "The name is Ike. Ike is here and he sends you his love." I just let out a big smile, and I said, "I know who you're talking about." Dwight's daughter always called him Ike, and his family called him Ike, and I always called him Dwight because I wasn't family. I guess this made me family.

When you asked Dwight or Ike to be your guardian angel, did you do that spontaneously, or had you thought about that ahead of time?

No, it just came to me to do that. I had never asked anybody to be my guardian angel, but I just felt that something special was needed. I wanted to give him a purpose, or something that he could do for me. I knew that this was a very important thing to do at that time. Even though I told him, "Dwight, nobody could ever replace you; you're just too special," I still had to give him more; it wasn't enough. So the guardian angel request just came out.

It was really a powerful relationship, and I'm not sure how it developed. It just happened; I let it happen. I wasn't forceful. I wasn't there asking 50 million questions and trying to keep him busy that way. I just felt what was in my heart and said it to him.

5 UNCONDITIONAL LOVE IN A CATASTROPHIC WORLD

It is no exaggeration to say that some old men and women live in a catastrophic world. They feel helpless, without value, and alone. This attitude cannot be dismissed as neurotic or unrealistic. In point of fact, they have lost many of their personal and social resources, have little control over their immediate environment, and face a future (if they can bring themselves to think about it) in which more loss and peril await. The massive dislocation, disorientation, and stunned response of the victim of a natural disaster has a close parallel in the geriatric patient, although the catastrophe in this case is individual and therefore more likely to escape general notice (Kastenbaum, 1964).

Care-givers are likely to feel as overmatched as the infirm and vulnerable aged themselves. What can be done realistically to compensate for the losses that have been suffered? It is no wonder that physicians, psychologists, nurses—even ministers—have hesitated to involve themselves intimately in what appears to be a losing cause.

Yet intimate involvement could well be the key. As the therapy program established itself, those of us who were in the roles of supervisors and enablers were impressed by the ability of the therapists to create intimate, shared worlds with people who had seemed doomed to isolation because of their severe impairments. This first of two commentary chapters tries to put the involvement and sharing process into focus.

181

LOVE, SUGGESTION, AND
"GETTING THROUGH"

How are the therapists themselves to be described? They are young people with undergraduate degrees who came to Cushing Hospital with the essential personality characteristics already well developed. If we tried to list these characteristics, they would certainly include a high level of empathy, the desire to help others, and the willingness to give fully of themselves. Furthermore, they have absolute respect and unconditional positive regard for all individuals. They see each person as unique, unlike any other. Is this a recital of cliches? No. These are the actual characteristics that all the therapists have in common—their defining characteristics, in fact.

If there is any secret to successful therapy with severely impaired geriatric patients, it is to be found in the life philosophy and personality strengths of the therapists themselves. Issues of technique are relevant and will be discussed. We would go amiss, however, if technique were emphasized to the neglect of the strengths of the individuals who themselves found the way to establish and maintain intimate human relationship under extremely difficult circumstances.

A wide variety of therapeutic approaches are used, some of which are unusual, original, and, often enough, impromptu as well. They demonstrate again that therapy is a living process, not a logico-deductive or cookbook system. Each therapist feels free to be herself and to approach each situation with spontaneity as well as a sense of its relationship to what has gone before.

All the therapeutic relationships, however, appear to draw upon the same fundamental orientation. We have found no better term for this than *unconditional love*. By this term we mean that the therapist truly loves and respects the patient, has no behavioral criteria upon which her love and respect are contingent, and does not hesitate to convey this to the patient. This is diametrically opposite to behavior modification approaches in which rewards or reinforcements are paid out to the patient only when the terms of a contract are met. The patients in our clinical program received everything the therapists had to offer—regardless.

Unconditional love is similar as a philosophy of care to what Carl Rogers has termed "unconditional positive regard" (Rogers, 1951).

The difference resides in the intense and encompassing nature of the relationship needed by and provided to these lonely and disabled patients. It is possible that Rogers himself, faced with the desperate situation of these geriatric patients, would also have spontaneously touched, hugged, and kissed as a natural part of his relationship-building. "Unconditional love therapy" (if such a term can be countenanced) has the aspect of Rogerian unconditional positive regard turned up to the highest notch. The positive regard cannot be communicated over a desk or by words alone. Instead, it must be made manifest so clearly, so directly, so imaginatively, and so persistently that the patient at last can again trust the good intentions of the world and value his or her own self.

Another prevalent aspect in this therapy program is the extensive use of suggestions. These are sincere and natural, not contrived in the seminar room and applied mechanically. The suggestions are nonverbal as well as verbal, indirect as well as direct.

Still a third major aspect is the therapist's ability to make contact. Many of the patients included in this program had been considered disoriented, out of contact, unable to understand or respond. For this reason, attention will also be given in the following case commentaries to the process of "getting through" and bridging what often seemed to be unbrigeable interpersonal gaps.

The following case comments exemplify the importance and prevalence of unconditional love, the use of suggestions, and the process of establishing a shared world.

CASE COMMENTS

Ginger S. came to Cushing Hospital after fifteen years of institutionalization, accompanied by a record that stated she was totally blind, deaf, and unable to communicate. This reputation could have served as a self-fulfilling prophecy. It implied that there was not much point in trying to communicate with Ginger or expecting much from her, thereby drawing the net of isolation even more tightly around her. Yet, this woman seems to have been a wife and mother of three children, a woman who coped adequately with life until her seventies. Perhaps being placed in a state hospital was such a disruptive and unacceptable experience to her that Ginger literally shut her eyes and ears to her new environment, and kept them closed when she was transferred to Cushing as well.

Beverly may well have been the first person in years to make a serious and systematic attempt to communicate with her. Beverly approached Ginger as if she could hear and see, at least a little. Nevertheless, Beverly emphasized touch: "I approached Ginger very gently and touched her on the shoulder and patted her, held her hand." Even a person totally blind and deaf can respond to affectionate touch. As Beverly made progress with Ginger, it became apparent that she did have some sight and hearing, although both senses were impaired. Aware of Ginger's visual limitations, Beverly chose a birthday card with embossed flowers. She enhanced the sensory allure of this card by scenting it with perfume, and then had Ginger smell the flowers and trace them with her fingers. This maximized Ginger's experience of the card by adding the less impaired modalities of smell and touch to her impaired sight. Within two weeks of the first contact, there was a dramatic change in Ginger. She stopped trembling when people approached and could now be described as "serene and relaxed." After fifteen years or more, someone had reached out to Ginger and conveyed concern for her as a person. This is probably why she could relax: she felt safe.

It is characteristic of Beverly and the other therapists to speak to their patients as though they are capable of understanding—if not all the words, then, at least, something of the tone and intent. An outsider might well have been astonished to overhear Beverly speaking of philosophical concerns to an old woman with expressive aphasia and many other disabilities. Beverly did not condescend, patronize, or trivialize. She respected Ginger as an intelligent adult although fully recognizing that she is also suffering serious impairments.

Ginger was one of the first patients seen in this therapy program, and she drew from Beverly a type of response that occurred again and again with other patients and other therapists. At one point, Ginger was perilously ill. She "began to have a difficult time breathing. I got even closer to her, almost held her, told her, It's all right, I'm here. It's all right! For maybe fifteen minutes, maybe half an hour. It was as if time were suspended. There was nothing but myself and Ginger."

This was a highly significant interaction. Many other individuals might have shied away from a person suffering acute respiratory distress. It is a distressful scene to witness. Beverly came even closer.

She continually assured Ginger that "it's all right!" What does this mean? The situation was anything but "all right." Ginger, already a severely debilitated person, was in the midst of a physiological crisis. What was the "it" and how could "it" be "all right"?

We believe the answer is implicit in remarks by Lawrence LeShan during a presentation he made to the CH staff. LeShan, a pioneer in psychotherapy with people suffering from life-threatening illness, gave several illustrations of the "it's okay" response. One example will suffice here. A child cries out in fear at night. One of the parents enters the room and judges that the child has had a nightmare. "It's okay," reassures the parent and sits for a moment hugging the child. Episode resolved. The "it" is nothing less than the entire world as perceived. The world had turned frightening. The parent's touch, proximity, and redefinition of the situation ("It's okay") restores a sense of basic security. And yet, as the parent walks back down the steps, he or she knows very well that it is not really that okay. The world is truly a frightening and insecure place at times, and it cannot be made entirely okay for children no matter how one tries.

The CH therapists often spontaneously provided this sense of comfort in a troubled world. "It's okay" statements are found in many transcripts prior to as well as following LeShan's talk. This reassurance probably would have had little effect with Ginger or other patients if it had not arisen within a deeply caring relationship. Among the cases reported in this book, "It's okay's" appear in the transcripts of Leonard R., George L., Doris G., Robin J., Maria F., and Matilda D., as well as Ginger S. It is possible that the therapists are confirming their own faith and comforting themselves as well as the patient when they say, "It's okay." This little phrase represents a sense of basic trust and confidence within a world that otherwise could be felt as catastrophic. The roots of this expression perhaps can be found in early mother–infant closeness, but the flowering also requires a seasoned optimism that comes with emotional maturity.

Beverly's relationship with Ginger did not keep the traditional "professional distance." She wept not only when Ginger died but also for the losses she had experienced during her life (for example, "the years she had been institutionalized, the years she had no one to relate to . . ."). Beverly even dreamed of Ginger and did not hesitate to share this dream with her. Ginger's eyes "filled up and she patted" Beverly's hand when hearing of the dream in which Ginger was healthy, standing up, and beautiful. This "dream gift" was entirely natural within the intimate relationship that had been established, and examples of this kind occurred with other therapists and other patients. Professional distance is an important concept, and one not to be set aside lightly. Nevertheless, it appears obvious that intimacy and empathy to the point of vulnerability on the part of the therapist have been keys to creating a helping relationship with seriously impaired old men and women.

Robin J., although a distinct individual, typifies the old person who has been left with extensive brain damage after multiple strokes. Her problems were compounded by aphasia. Beverly bridged the communication gap by gentle, caring touch, positive suggestions, and reassurance. These are essentially simple and obvious actions, and yet Robin had been deprived of such interactions for a long time. The ideas that Robin was still a worthwhile person and could still participate pleasurably in life were astounding. They seemed so out of keeping with the poor quality of life she had been experiencing.

Unfortunately, it is natural to limit our verbal interaction with aphasic patients. Certainly, it is rare to "converse" with an old woman who herself cannot speak; yet this is done routinely by the CH therapists. Beverly, for instance, is able to feel comfortable with a monologue—and yet, when we look closely, we see that Robin is participating. This takes place because Beverly is carefully observing Robin's nonverbal reactions and works these into her conversation. This acute awareness of the patient's nonverbal responses enables the therapists to feel reinforced by the slightest response. They do not fall into the trap of assuming the patient is unaware and nonresponsive just because no words are forthcoming.

When Beverly explains brain damage and its effects to Robin, she is treating her as an intelligent person with the right to know what has happened to her. Again, this is a simple and obvious action, and again, it is an action that is seldom taken with people in Robin's situation. Even if Robin is unable to comprehend all the technicalities of what Beverly is telling her, she still feels and understands the intent of the explanation as well as the respect Beverly has for her intelligence and her being. "Little" thoughts open new vistas. For example, Beverly "spoke of the spring and coming to the garden...." We can speculate that this was the first time *in years* that anyone had suggested to Robin that there still was a possibility that she might be able to do something—that she might be able to see a garden again— and that her life was not completely over.

Exemplifying the therapists' devotion to their patients is the following: Beverly left her own family to come in for a few hours on Christmas Day to feed Robin her dinner and give her a present. She selected a brightly colored shawl, knowing, from her observations, that Robin enjoys bright colors.

The therapists have also made themselves skilled in identifying and encouraging their patients' positive experiences. For instance, when Beverly asked Robin to try writing something, she immediately became aware of her disappointment that she could only turn out scribbles. Beverly quickly reinterpreted Robin's failure (to write words) as a success (holding and moving a pen again).

Beverly and the other therapists often are with the patient, whenever possible, at the time of death. Their comforting presence is felt by any relatives who might be present, as was the case with Robin, as well as by the patients themselves. We believe the death-bed comfort provided by the therapists is appreciated by the nursing staff as well. It underlines the importance of what they have been doing to provide care and comfort. There are extended care facilities where patients are "dropped" when death is in prospect: "There's nothing more we can do! There's nothing more we should do!" The fact that somebody who doesn't *have* to be on the ward (the therapist) chooses to be there as the patient is dying is an affirmation that what the nurses are doing to provide care is also important because the dying person is still important.

George L. presented a different set of problems. His manic behavior was difficult for staff to manage. It was recognized that the manic high was part of a cycle he had been going through for many years, but this did not make management any easier. George was described as "racing around the hospital, confused, difficult to manage, and voiding where he shouldn't." This type of behavior poses a considerable challenge within the open environment of CH, a facility designed for people who are in control of themselves. We would not put a person such as George in a locked ward—there are no locked wards at Cushing—nor would we subject him to heavy medication. This means that no simple and automatic solutions are available.

Beverly was able to form a therapeutic alliance with George by recognizing that his agitated behavior was more than a conventional manic attack. She understood that it was related to the fear of dying that had preoccupied him since age sixteen and was now aggravated by a bronchial condition. With this understanding and her character-istic rich empathy, Beverly was able to avoid treating George as a "disruptive behavior problem" (although he was, in fact, a source of disruption within the hospital). This means that she did not have to position herself defensively and wrestle with George to make him manageable. Instead, she truly felt for him: "It's hard for me to talk about this, because I'm feeling so much of what he must have been experiencing." With this approach, there was no tug of wills between therapist and patient. Despite his state of fear, agitation, and confu-sion, George quickly recognized that Beverly was on his side.

In relating to George, Beverly accepted him, religious preoccupa-tions and all. The most common response to George and other agi-tated people with dominating religious ideology is to avoid and ignore this subject. She went right to it, and this seemed to be an important factor in creating a shared world. Once admitted to this world, Beverly was able to endow it with a more serene and positive ambiance. She helped George use his own religious beliefs to control his fears, replacing an angry, vengeful God with a God of "love, peace, and forgiveness." From a technical standpoint, it might be said that the therapist identified and accepted the patient's own con-struct system (Kelly 1955), and then used this indigenous system to generate the positive suggestions. This is as different as can be from a therapist marching in with a set of prepared suggestions that are alien to the particular client's phenomenological framework.

Once the relationship settled in, Beverly taught George to relax. This action immediately demonstrated to George that he could have favorable influence over his own state of mind. It also indicated to the staff that George was teachable and not entirely a passive victim of manic attacks. The secure relationship between patient and thera-pist also took some of the pressure off the ward staff who know they can always call on Beverly to reinforce her previous work with him by further relaxation exercises and assurances that he will be all right.

Deep relaxation and guided imagery techniques were effectively combined in Beverly's work with John Z. More interesting than the techniques per se, however, was the challenge that confronted the therapist and the distinctive interpersonal climate among ward staff. Gangrene is a difficult and often frustrating condition for the nursing staff to treat. Apart from specific problems in providing effective treatment, the staff must adjust to the sight and odor of dying tissue.

Beverly had to overcome her own horrified reaction to the condition of John's legs ("There were many wide areas of black, and there was stuff oozing out. A part of me said, 'Oh God, what can be done? And another part of me became transformed.") She recognized her conflicted feelings, then relaxed "and felt confident that something could be done." Her confidence seemed to depend, however, on whether Beverly relied more on her logic or her feelings ("If I were going to be logical, then I had to wonder if anything could be done."). This kind of ambivalence has been experienced by many people who are on the threshold of forming a therapeutic relationship. Those who draw back often can find ample justification in the apparent facts of the situation. Beverly, like the other therapists in this program, clearly recognized the formidable realities but stepped forward anyway.

The situation was made exceptional by the fact that the nursing staff on this ward shares the philosophy of life that is known as Charismatic Christianity. This includes belief in the efficacy of faith healing (but it also includes belief in the efficacy of good nursing and medical care). Beverly was welcome in this group, as evidenced by the circle of prayer they spontaneously formed together. Therapy with John Z. could call upon an interpersonal atmosphere of positive suggestion and belief, and therefore was perhaps this program's closest parallel to some of the healing environments that were described in the historical survey. But therapy with John Z. also meant the challenge of trying to prevent gangrene-instigated amputation, a major physical problem.

The successful outcome resulted from a team effort, in which the provision of dedicated nursing care was an indispensable element. Beverly was not a healer working in isolation from the basic ward staff and accomplishing what they could not. Instead, she was able to form an effective therapeutic alliance that helped John himself to become a major factor in his own recovery. She wasted no time in making it clear to John that he himself had the power to exercise a positive influence over his body. She did not make the process appear exotic or arcane. Instead, Beverly patiently explained to John something of the way in which the body's own healing process works. This simple and common-sense explanation also served to locate John and Beverly's efforts together within the broader context of the medical and nursing care that was being offered.

This was another relationship in which the therapist dreamed of the patient as a healthy, whole person. In sharing this dream with John, Beverly was also conveying the implicit suggestion that he *can* be healed, making her dream come true.

At least one another "little thing" should be mentioned. Geriatric patients often have their lives narrowed by illness and hospitalization. Concern becomes focused on the self, and understandably so. John, however, reached the point where he spontaneously asked Beverly how *she* was. Although still cognitively impaired (for instance, unable to remember names), he has become interested in the people who have become interested in him. This is not a negligible development; it represents a tide of human concern and empathy passing back and forth, instead of a perpetual giver matched to a perpetual receiver.

STARTING THE RELATIONSHIP

It is worth focusing on the early stages of therapy. Many of the old men and women had become increasingly isolated over months, years, even decades. Whatever might have been the original context of isolation, these people were now further handicapped by a variety of perceptual and cognitive disabilities. How did the therapists establish contact?

Maria F. was on a trajectory that could have led to rapid decline and death. She was refusing all food and drink, and she never spoke. Additionally, her native language was Italian, and apparently she did not have much English at her disposal. Judy literally reached out and touched Maria, holding her hand and speaking gently so that her intent if not the substance of her words might come across. Maria did understand that Judy was there to help her and would often be by her side. On some level, Maria came to expect and accept Judy's visits. Time began to mean something again; there was something worthwhile to expect. As simple as it seems, this revitalization of time probably was important to Maria and many other isolated individuals in providing them with an alternative to the extremely private, unconnected world they had been inhabiting. The symbolic link between private and shared world was as palpable as Judy's hand in hers. Once Judy had been admitted to the threshold of Maria's world, it was then possible for further progress to be made.

Early in the relationship, Judy did two things that are typical of the therapists: she imagined herself being in the patient's situation, and she relieved some of the patient's anxiety by explanations. After empathically placing herself in Maria's situation, Judy could perceive certain sounds and events as threatening (the squeaking wheels on an unseen attendant's cart passing in the hall; the sudden and mysterious noise that was nothing more than a toilet being flushed). Characteristically, the therapists make a point of trying to experience the world from the patient's perspective. This often enables them to make useful guesses about sources of anxiety and stress and to come up with ways to enrich a deprived life space.

Time and again, the therapists do that little something extra that improves the possibility of starting a relationship. When Beverly first saw Helen C., for example, she was careful to align her own head with the patient's to achieve eye contact. This was accompanied by a friendly touch and asking the patient if she could come to visit. Residents of institutions (not only of geriatric institutions) seldom have their opinions and preferences consulted. Beverly and the other therapists often ask permission and then honor the patient's response. This simple procedure helps the patient to feel more like a normal human being whose preferences matter. It also helps to reestablish the self as a center of control. Discouraged and alienated geriatric patients may seek to exercise control by refusing to take nourishment or resisting other procedures. When the patient is clearly treated with respect and asked rather than told to do things, then the need for inappropriate demonstrations of control lessens.

Alfred B. was suffering acutely from his lack of understanding of an environmental change when Lisa was first asked to work with him. It is almost certain that nurses had told Alfred he would be moved temporarily to another ward in the same hospital while his own ward was being painted. He did not retain this information, however, and found the move quite disruptive, the problems intensified by his blindness. Before Lisa could establish any kind of relationship with him, she had to look past his belligerent demeanor. She recognized that Alfred was being "tough" and combative because he really felt alone and threatened. He could account for the upsetting change only by supposing that some kind of conspiracy was at work ("This is a murder house. . . . The doctor gives you poison pills."). Lisa was not frightened or put off by this behavior. Instead, she gave him long, gentle backrubs as a concrete way of demonstrating her affection for him. The touching itself helped to circumvent Alfred's overheated verbal system, and the fact that she gave him a long, lingering backrub helped him to realize that Lisa was not simply doing a job that she had to do as quickly as possible. The backrubs became a nightly ritual, providing Alfred with a core of stability around which he could reorganize himself. The trust that Alfred was able to develop toward Lisa soon spread to include other staff and the new ward in general.

Lisa's work with Alfred exemplifies another feature that has often emerged. It turned out that Alfred could hear and comprehend more than had been supposed, and that his "bizarre, inappropriate" behavior was serving a purpose for him (keeping a threatening world away). Through their sensitivity and respect, the therapists have found that even quite debilitated or confused patients often have more assets than they have been credited with. Sometimes these assets have been concealed as part of a defensive strategy, at other times they have been unavailable to the patients themselves until facilitated by a caring relationship.

BEDSIDE PHILOSOPHY

Some of the most significant therapeutic developments have been associated with an approach that has little currency in contemporary practice and which might appear totally inappropriate with severely disabled geriatric patients. Philosophical discourse has been supplanted by many other therapeutic modes. It is part of the intellectualization that psychodynamic theorists perceive as defensive and which constitutes irrelevant verbal output for the behaviorists. This lack of confidence in a philosophical approach is not capricious. Philosophy can, in fact, be defensive intellectualization on part of both therapist and client. Furthermore, the relationships between verbal concepts, inner experience, and behavior are variable and complex. There is ample justification for therapists to pay attention, as they do, to much more than philosophy.

Advanced age has often been considered a contraindication for any type of psychological therapy. "Talking philosophy" with geriatric patients perhaps qualifies as the most unlikely approach of all. They would not understand philosophical issues because of cognitive deficits and perhaps the relatively low formal educational level of people in the present generations of the aged. Furthermore, even if they did understand, such abstract discussion would seem irrelevant because they are afflicted with so many very practical and immediate problems. And, if we require still another negative, even if the debilitated old could understand philosophy and find it relevant, why should we suppose that philosophical discourse should have any discernible effect?

With this kind of background expectation in mind, one would have to be surprised at what actually has been happening in a number of therapist–patient interactions. One particularly clear example occurred with Rose T., an eighty-seven-year-old woman whose case has not previously been reported. If it is proper to speak of types of people, then there are thousands of Rose T.'s around the nation. These are the people found on the back wards of mental institutions or in any facility where nature and society's failures are housed out of sight. This is the person who has had serious emotional disturbances in early adulthood and whose treatment has gradually became more and more of the problem itself. Specifically, she is a victim of tardive dyskinesia, a condition for which no successful treatment is known and which itself is produced by years of high-dosage antipsychotic medication. The symptoms of tardive dyskinesia include characteristic grimaces, posturing, and tongue movements as well as probable additional brain damage. All of these problems, added to the difficulties the person had already been carrying, make the individual appear almost a caricature of a normal human being. It takes a rather special nursing staff to provide alert and faithful care; one's first impulse is to shrink away from what seems a frightening example of how much can go wrong with the human condition.

Rose T. had been receiving good nursing care at Cushing, but was locked in one of her periodic catatonic states, not responding to the environment and becoming combative when approached. Beverly started working regularly *not* with Rose but with a neighboring patient for whom she had received a consult. In the style that is natural to her, Beverly would often discuss philosophical, meaning-of-life matters with the other patient. Rose was listening all the time! These discussions seemed to stimulate a woman who for fifty-five years had been withdrawn into her own world.

To Beverly's amazement, Rose suddenly "came to life" and asked, "Who are you?" Beverly told her that she was a therapist who was here because she loved and cared for people. There was another and even more surprising question. Rose wanted to know *why*. She wanted to know why we come into this world, live a few years, suffer so much of the time, and then die.

How would a traditional therapist respond to this question, especially coming from a debilitated old woman with a long and continuing history of psychosis? Would not the question most likely have been side-stepped in some way, gotten around, converted into something else?

Beverly, who knew nothing about Rose and her background, responded spontaneously that she has suffered in her life, too. Since she has had to suffer, Beverly has tried to learn from it. Perhaps, Beverly suggested, I can help you to learn from the kind of suffering you yourself have been experiencing. And then, when the moment seemed right, Beverly added, "But I don't think it is meant that you suffer anymore. It seems to me that you have done your share of suffering." An extended conversation followed. It would have been remarkable enough to have a genuine conversation with Rose on any subject. But the subject here was nothing less than the meaning of life. Rose confided that her main concern over all these years has been to try to understand why her life has come to this, why she seemed destined to live and die in an institution. Beverly's impulse was to hug her and cry her heart out. Instead, she answered that she didn't know the reason either, repeating her thought that all this suffering had been more than eough and that it could now come to an end. (The hug did come, later, as Beverly left for the day.) There was additional discussion of life and suffering. Having Rose's full attention, Beverly placed a positive suggestion with her: "Something new and wonderful is going to open up for you and you will experience happiness—and your happiness will mean so much more because of all your suffering."

At a check point four months after this breakthrough, the head nurse reported a remarkable improvement for Rose. After another month, Rose was up and around the hospital—for the first time ever—and had even been out for a drive for the first time in fifty years. "Beverly is my loyal, faithful friend," she tells everybody. Gone are her former frequent night terrors about the devils who were coming to get her.

This development would probably have been impossible if the ward staff had not continued to maintain Rose's health over a long period of time and to provide her with an objectively (if not subjectively) secure environment. Beverly's intervention demonstrated the value of something we have already described in other instances, the use of strong positive suggestions within an intensely caring relationship. But it also demonstrates that philosophical discourse can be powerful at the bedside of that seemingly most unlikely candidate, the debilitated geriatric patient. We suggest that one of the reasons for this improbable outcome is quite a simple one: the questions we call philosophic are not at all abstract for such a person. The meaning of life and death, of suffering and loss—such questions are not academic exercises here, nor facile evasions of deeper, underlying problems. Life, death, suffering, and loss are right there, most palpably. Rose T. had every reason to be involved in a philosophical quest, and without someone such as Beverly on the scene, she might have continued to the end of her life without ever sharing her concern. How many other Rose T.'s are there?

Philosophical and, one must add, *spiritual* concerns often are discussed as a natural part of therapy at Cushing Hospital. Matilda D., for example, was much attuned to the subjects of God and nature, subjects that are also close to Andrea. This shared universe of concern helped them swiftly establish an intimate relationship that was a source of comfort for Matilda as her life neared its end.

Praying together is not usually found in the approved list of therapeutic techniques, but has proven natural and effective in some cases. This is illustrated by Lisa's work with Bonita A., a woman born eighty-eight years ago in Italy. Bonita remained mentally alert and had good eyesight and hearing, but had discomfort from degenerative arthritis. She was receiving treatment for this distress, including hot packs from physical therapy, but continued to request (and receive) Codein, and feared that her pain might increase. She could stand up and ambulate short distances with a walker, but she preferred to stay in bed. Bonita was uncomfortable, anxious, participated little in activities and programs, did not make much use of her remaining physical capacities, and was described as a "difficult, demanding" patient.

She is now a "pleasant and cooperative person" who travels considerable distances with her walker and even takes a few steps on her own. Bonita crochets, knits, and makes handicraft items of high quality. She has pain at times in limited areas and of brief duration, seldom requesting medication. Bonita even looks different: her skin has cleared, is no longer tight and tender. The list of improvement goes on: better appetite, pleasurable participation in occupational therapy and recreational therapy, trips outside the hospital, and, not least, her own feeling that she is ten years younger and much happier.

What happened between "before" and "after"? The continuation of alert medical and nursing care kept Bonita in shape to benefit maximally from the relationship with Lisa. Much of what Lisa did has already been noted in other cases—establishing trust, conveying strong and unconditional affection, offering a series of positive suggestions, and teaching in positive self-suggestion. A long chapter could be devoted to the specific ways in which Lisa worked with Bonita to facilitate this notable physical, psychological, and social improvement. There was something more, however. Bonita and Lisa were compatible in their deep religious beliefs (as was true with Matilda and Andrea). Their shared philosophy of life was made manifest by praying together. It was further represented in overt action by therapeutic touch. For people with certain religious and spiritual orientations, the comfort of gentle touch from a caring person is augmented by the belief that a kind of healing energy is being transmitted. This was a shared belief for Bonita and Lisa. Whether or not there is something in nature that answers to the name of healing energy, the belief in such a benign force probably adds to the basic comfort of a caring relationship.

Praying and laying-on-of-hands with Bonita and Lisa, and other examples of philosophical and spiritual interactions are found in many, though by no means all, of the case records. It should be emphasized that these are not procedures that are administered or applied as self-contained strategies. Instead, they arise organically within the relationships. One should not expect to obtain the same results by simply walking up to a patient and touching, praying, or talking philosophy. Many interpersonal skills are involved, as well as the ability to give deeply of oneself.

OTHER DIMENSIONS

This chapter has considered some of the major dimensions of holistic therapy with the aged. There are many other dimensions, however, some of which raise difficult problems. This is why another chapter follows.

REFERENCE

Rogers, C. *Client-centered therapy.* Boston: Houghlin Mifflin, 1951.

6 TOWARD MORE EFFECTIVE THERAPY

Old. Sick. Helpless. These words describe most of the people served by our therapy program. It is obvious that at its most effective, our efforts did not reverse oldness. To be old is simply to have reached a station of psychobiological development. It is doubtful that being old is in itself a basis for initiating therapy. At every time of life a person can benefit from friendship and affection, but therapy is a different matter. Sickness is also a different matter. Much of what presents itself as the miseries of aging has to do with illness and functional impairment. The classic NIMH study (Birren, Butler, Greenhouse, Sokoloff, and Yarrow, 1963) made it clear that people who reach the later years of life free of illness also are free of many of the problems that are often thought of as intrinsic to aging. There are many men and women equivalent in age to Cushing Hospital patients who are doing quite well in the community. Being old presents unique challenges, but it is being sick that places the individual in serious peril.

Helplessness is both an objective and a subjective matter. To varying degrees, the person who has become an institutionalized geriatric patient has lost some of his or her ability to master the environment. A successful institutional arrangement provides such a person with an environment that is easier to manage, a small and predictable world in which one can function more effectively (less helplessly). The

197

sense of helplessness has a variable relationship to the person's actual ability to act effectively in the world. Some people quickly develop a massive sense of helplessness after a trauma, a loss, a failure. Even though they retain much coping ability, there is a dejection and lack of confidence that is nearly as debilitating as actual physical impairment. Others are more fortunate in being able to recognize their strengths as well as their handicaps and so to chart a reasonable course of action.

It is possible that the therapeutic program described here has played a role in alleviating some of the sickness and objective helplessness (ineffectiveness) that has clouded the lives of our patients. It is probable that the program has done much to help them overcome the sense of helplessness. We would like to believe that the therapeutic relationships have restored self-confidence and a species of hope. With this improved feeling about oneself and the world, perhaps favorable processes were stimulated, such as: (1) increased use of residual abilities that had been held back because of motivational and emotional factors; (2) relaxation and tension-reduction that make it easier for the natural healing functions of the body to succeed. Furthermore, family members and other staff may have been encouraged by the patients' response to therapy and consequently looked for new ways to make contributions themselves.

But is there justification for our impression of therapeutic efficacy? On the face of it, the program has been successful, with favorable outcomes continuing to be observed for many individuals beyond those described in this book. There is a difference, however, between impression and definitive knowledge. Firm and precise conclusions elude us, and we knew in advance that this would be the case. This chapter will explore what has been learned and what has yet to be learned about the effectiveness of such a therapeutic program with institutionalized geriatric patients. The decisions we have made—correctly or incorrectly—may themselves be of interest to others who are interested in providing care for people with such deep physical, psychological, and social needs. More importantly, whatever the actual effectiveness of what we have been doing up to this point, we have the responsibility to find ways to be of greater assistance in the future. This aim leads us through the varied topics that comprise this chapter.

THERAPY OR EVALUATION OF THERAPY?

Theoretically, one can both provide therapy and conduct appropriate evaluation of therapy. In practical terms, however, one sometimes has to choose. We thought first of doing both. With reluctance, we decided that the therapy itself would not have its best chance if saddled with the rigorous controls of a formal evaluation effort worthy of the name. We did not much care for the prospect of burdening the entire hospital, that complex and living organism, with an additional set of procedures and obligations on top of all the existing regulations and exigencies. Furthermore, we did not want to establish an apparatus that might give the appearance of systematic evaluation without the reality. The following considerations are among the many that lead us to forego formal evaluation.

1. *Therapist variables.* What the therapist does—and who the therapist *is*—obviously is part of the process. It is true that many studies evaluating psychotherapy have been conducted in essential ignorance of precisely what the therapists did and how they did it. We did not think it useful to add to this branch of the literature. The most commanding way to know what therapists do is first to specify their actions in advance and then monitor them as they go along. This strategy is not easy to apply in any situation, but is within reason when the therapeutic approach is of the behavioral modification type, and the situational context is fairly simple (for instance, the client appears in the therapist's office at scheduled intervals for specific help with specific problems). Such a strategy is admirable for evaluation purposes, but we judged it would have been misapplied here. We did not think it wise to specify in advance precisely what the therapists would and would not do. We could agree among ourselves on therapeutic philosophy and major techniques. There was not sufficient knowledge base, however, to give specific instructions to the therapists. This could only have placed them at a disadvantage as they encountered unique situations with individual patients. We could ask them to keep notes on every session and to discuss their work in detail with a supervisor, and these procedures were followed systematically. (The presentations to the listener which form the basis for the case histories in this book were over and above the basic reporting system.) More elaborate and complete documentation of

the therapeutic process could have been accomplished by videotaping sessions, but this technique seemed guaranteed to create unwanted difficulties for the new program.

We recognized that if the therapists were to have their necessary flexibility, then we could have only an approximate idea of what they would do until they had actually done it. This made it difficult to link treatment with outcome variables. One could examine simple and rather empty variables, for example, the number of sessions, but this would not likely tell us much about the therapeutic workings themselves. Furthermore, the matchup between therapist and client also presents another set of relevant variables. Any serious evaluation procedure would require a systematic therapist–assignment method. Otherwise it is virtually impossible to disentangle characteristics of a particular therapist from the approach in general and from the problems and strengths of a particular patient.

2. *Outcome variables.* Precisely what did we expect—or hope—that therapy might accomplish? In a general sense, of course, we would have counted therapy successful if the patients "got better" or "felt better." Being more specific about the possible outcomes was more difficult. Was it reasonable to expect therapy to have the same outcomes in all cases? For one person a renewal of social interest and activity might seem the most appropriate goal, while for another the ability to carry out even a little daily self-care might be a triumph. The level of possible outcome could vary greatly and would be difficult to compare. We did not anticipate, for example, that one man would be in danger of requiring double amputation and that therapy might contribute to his recovery without surgery. But we were aware that decubitis ulcers (bed sores) are fairly common among debilitated patients who spend much of their time in bed. Some people have decubiti at the time of admission; others suffer skin breakdown later despite attentive nursing care. If the healing tradition is to be taken seriously, then therapists with this gift might exercise some type of influence that results in self-repair of the lesion. But can the tradition be taken this seriously? Should we specify healing of these physical lesions as a reasonable outcome of therapy when we could not really specify the processes involved?

The questions go on. Has therapy been successful if the patient lives longer than expected? Or has it been successful if the patient comes to accept death with serenity? How are the various possible outcomes to be weighted—which changes are of most importance?

How do we compare a dramatic improvement that does not last with a lesser improvement that has staying power? Are the outcomes to be specified within the framework of the patient, family, therapist, or other staff members? The therapy program confirmed our earlier experiences in that the various people on the scene often had different outcome goals, certainly different priorities. Relative, nurse, and therapist, for example, all might feel that they know what the patient wants or what is best for the patient, and yet all have different goals in mind. The patient, whose own wishes were to be consulted and elicited whenever possible, would not always be in the position to give us clear direction.

Problems such as these could be reduced if one carefully controlled access to therapy. Only patients with the kind of problems whose treatment we could best evaluate might be accepted. One might, for example, select only those with decubiti, providing therapy for part of this subgroup while the others were in a no-treatment subgroup. However, any approach that established rigid prerequisites for therapy seemed unwise to us. Some patients whom the medical and nursing staff believed could benefit from therapy might be excluded, while others might be assigned to therapy against the judgment of staff. We judged it more sensible to have referrals become part of the hospital flow rather than institute a rigid selection process that was likely to create difficulties and then falter without achieving its objective.

3. *Contextual variables.* The shifting realities of the hospital situation (and, indeed, of the general socioeconomic climate that influences staff and family as well as patients) exercise influence over the treatment process. These variables are hard enough just to catalog, let alone index and assess. A few of the variables can be manipulated, but most are beyond the reach of research. The therapy program as a program itself influences the situational context which simultaneously welcomes, resists, and ignores the new program. With blinders in place we might attend only to what transpires between patient and therapist. It is obvious, however, that the patient's mood of the moment, the therapist's sense of being welcomed or resented on the ward, and many other factors in the situational swirl do influence the therapeutic process.

Consider one of the many types of contextual variables at work: staff coverage. Providing adequate nursing coverage throughout the twenty-four-hour day requires close monitoring and frequent readjustment. The number of personnel, their level of training and experience, and their familiarity with particular patients all vary over time. This means that potentially important differences might well occur in the pattern of nursing care for a given patient, differences that could obscure the possible impact of therapy. A related variable, ward climate, also varies over time and makes it difficult to assess therapy-related outcome with any precision.

For reasons such as these, we decided to focus our energies on the therapy program itself. We judged that we could not put into place an apparatus that would both be successful as evaluation and responsive to hospital needs and realities. This meant that we would try to learn rather than prove or disprove. Our early experiences with the program subsequently could be put to use in designing relevant types of evaluation.

IN THE JUDGMENT OF OTHERS

How does the therapy program look to other staff members? Key staff with long experience at the hospital and no direct link to the program were asked for their observations. Interviews were conducted with staff well respected for their competence, commitment to patient care, and independence of mind. By the time of these interviews, the staff had had more than a year to witness and interact with the therapy program. What follows is the gist of these observations. We think they hold some instruction not only for improving one-to-one therapy in a particular geriatric facility but also for introducing and refining treatment programs of various types within complex settings.

William A. Richards, M.D., the medical director for more than a decade, consulted his records to check on sixty-four patients seen by Ryder and Doran. He considered himself sufficiently informed to make a judgment in fifty-five cases.

> In thirty-one of fifty-five I judged there was probable benefit from the supportive therapy. In twenty-four of fifty-five I recognized no effects not attributable to the patient's recognized diseases and other therapies. I recognized no cases wherein supportive therapy had been harmful to the patient.
>
> Therefore, I repeat my observation that one-to-one supportive therapy by psychology-trained persons under appropriate direction provides significant benefit to our patients. Also, I can identify no harmful effects.

There are two points of particular interest here. If there had been perception of harmful effects attributable to the therapy program, then the medical director and his staff would not have waited to be asked. We would have heard promptly. The same holds true for the nursing staff. As will be seen below, there were indeed some problems perceived by nursing personnel, but these were essentially of an organizational and interpersonal nature. If the therapists were having adverse effects on their patients, we would not have required retrospective surveys or statistical analyses to learn them; concerned staff would have expressed themselves in a vigorous wave of protest. The lack of staff-perceived negative effects is not the same as demonstration of the positive. However, this does remind us that in a complex real-life situation, such as a geriatric hospital, there are natural consequences that indicate how a particular program is faring.

The other point concerns the framework of evaluation. Every person with clinical responsibilities functions with inner guidelines and expectations which are applied constantly. Is this patient taking too long to recover from an infection? Has a certain standard of care been neglected with that patient? How was this other patient able to snap back from what ordinarily would have been a catastrophic illness? Each staff member has his or her own framework, shaped by experience, that is matched against actual observations. And this is perhaps the most significant testing process. A clinician well experienced with geriatric patients may read research findings with interest, but will probably depend on his or her own framework of judgment when making decisions or evaluating outcomes. It would be worth comparing analytically the diverse frameworks that guide each staff member. But it is also worth something to know that the therapy program registered as worthwhile within the everyday framework employed by a person with the perspective of the medical director.

Richards himself likens the problem of evaluating one-to-one therapy outcomes with the more general problem of evaluating *any* therapy outcome:

> For example, there are a multiplicity of things going on that affect the outcome of drug therapies, and I'm not speaking necessarily of psychotropic drugs. The evaluation of cause and effect in just about any area I can think of remains fraught with great peril. The fact that an area is "hard" or "soft" should not dissuade one from undertaking therapy, however. Except in massive statistical study as in epidemiological public health, this sort of evaluation stands very little chance of becoming completely well established. I

don't know how you could design a study to prove to everyone's satisfaction that this type of intervention is a grand and good thing!

He adds: "Certainly, no one has ever been able to prove to everyone's satisfaction that medicine itself is a grand and good thing!"

Judith Adam, then the senior supervisor of nurses, is a person with almost two decades of experience at Cushing Hospital. She pointed out situational problems as the program began.

> There was a lot of negative feeling (on the part of nursing) because we were so short in nursing and you were taking positions from nursing, although we really didn't lose attendants because of it, and I don't think there was a full understanding of what you were trying to do.

Nursing coverage was short during this period, just as Adam reports, and the supportive therapists were given job-blocks that "belonged" to nursing. This was done simply because there were no other blocks available for this purpose. Senior personnel had been informed that this assignment of positions would in no way detract from efforts to recruit more nursing staff at all levels of vacancy. The objective fact was that all suitable candidates were hired, with none turned away because therapists were now also on the staff. However, some ward staff came to the quick conclusion that the new therapists were "instead of," not "in addition to," and reacted adversely, as Adam noted.

She emphasized the staff's initial unfamiliarity with both the aims and techniques of the therapy program. Some of the negativity came from the unknowns that had been introduced. This was gradually alleviated as therapy supervisors described the program to the head nurses and conducted seminars that explicated their concepts and techniques. The unknowns gradually became more understandable and therefore acceptable. Furthermore, the nurses how had a clearer idea of whom to see and how to proceed if any problems developed with a particular case. The lines of authority and communication had not been clear enough at the beginning.

Adam voiced a concern that was felt by many nursing personnel at Cushing Hospital—the pressure to keep the basic, everyday things under control while still welcoming and participating in programs that might move us ahead. Those with the most intense pressure to meet problems of the moment tend to be impatient with any new development that does not seem to address the needs that are right in front of them. This assures a certain level of tension and conflict, especially at the early stages of a new program. Adam could see both sides of the situation. She empathized with ward staff in their concern for the basics, yet recognized that one-to-one relationships are also basic and should be provided in one way or another. She reminded the listener that the present department of recreation therapy was launched by a former CH nurse who developed this alternative method of providing social relationships and life enrichment to the patients.

From the perspective of this experienced nurse, then, one-to-one therapy and other types of interpersonal relationships definitely were needed to improve the patients' quality of life. It was not an easy thing, however, to balance this somewhat less traditional program with the evident and persistent needs for basic nursing care. She had respect and affection for the therapists themselves. One of her major concerns was for the emotional vulnerability of therapists who become so intensely involved with the patients. She did not see anything wrong with intense involvements per se, but suggested that ways be found to share the load and support the therapists themselves.

The issues identified by Adam were also brought out by most of the other interviewees and by other staff who volunteered observations from time to time. This includes the touchy question of who should "get credit" for therapeutic success. Any display on the part of the therapists that they considered themselves prime movers in successful outcomes would anger and alienate other staff. A spontaneous expression of pleasure on the part of a therapist as, for example, when a previously mute patient speaks her first words, could easily be interpreted as egotism. Few things could upset other staff members more than for therapists to give the impression that they had worked magic, had accomplished something that others could or did not. Adam's own position was that "I don't think that's important—who did it—just as long as the patient improved, and the one-to-one therapists can take just as much credit as nursing, recreation therapy, occupational therapy, and physical therapy can. It's team work, all of us working in the interests of the patient." This sentiment was expressed by the other interviewees as well.

Two other nursing supervisors also shared their views. Carol Gaudette, another person with many years of direct care experience at Cushing Hospital and current supervisor of the rehabilitation unit, emphasized the importance of team work, to which the one-to-one therapists were a welcome addition. The integration of therapists into the clinical team could have been quicker and smoother if there had been more discussion with the head nurses before the program started. Some of the therapists were more adept than others in making themselves part of the mainstream treatment pattern. One therapist, for example, often asked nursing for information and advice and in return gave them good feedback on her work with the patients. Another therapist, however, tended to act too independently, and this lead to several problems that could have been avoided with better communication. There are technical details in the care of geriatric patients that nurses can share with the therapists and which the therapists should be open to receive.

Gaudette is curious about the processes by which not only the therapists but nurses and other people are able to help debilitated patients. Current knowledge takes us only so far. In the case of John Z., for example, the nurses employed certain positioning techniques to increase circulation to his legs and were especially attentive to the dressing techniques used. These are overt, visible actions that probably contributed to his recovery. Yet Gaudette does not want to deny that Ryder may have contributed on a level that is just as real but less visible and more difficult to trace. "Maybe she did get across to his brain cells, through the barrier of chronic brain syndrome. Who's saying that this didn't help, how can you prove that?"

In company with the other respondents, Gaudette has become increasingly interested in the unknowns of health care, the ways in which one person can affect another for better or worse. The therapy program has helped to rekindle this interest. An unanticipated (though logical) outcome of the therapy program has been the arousal of curiosity and re-evaluation on the part of staff members who had become somewhat settled in their ways. The long-term effects of this spinoff could be interesting because Gaudette and others bring years of pragmatic experience to the analysis of new developments.

Cathy Mooney, another supervisor, first heard about the therapy program at staff conferences. This introduction was not enough to give her a firm understanding of the program, and her first reaction was negative "because my concern at the time was the lack of staff nursing. We were having a hard time meeting the patients' basic needs such as washing and dressing and ambulating, so it was kind of a negative attitude, I would say. I didn't really understand." It seemed to Mooney then that the hospital was investing in something else instead of basic patient care and this could only stir up negative feelings in her. "They were all upset because they were looking for more staff to take care of the basic needs of the patients rather than someone coming in 'just' sitting and talking to a patient." Many of the ward staff felt the same way.

This impression changed as she had the opportunity to meet the therapists and see them at work. The same is true for many of the ward staff now. She cited by way of example a current case in which Judy Doran has formed a therapeutic relationship with a man afflicted with a neurological condition that keeps him in almost constant distress. Doran takes him for long walks and gives him emotional support and companionship. Along with a careful medication program, this is probably what is responsible for the marked improvement the patient has been showing.

"I would like to see the supportive therapy continued," Mooney declared. She would also like for nursing personnel to have more opportunity both to learn and perform these functions themselves. A number of nurses and attendants have expressed an interest in doing so since they have witnessed the therapy program at work. The communication and education programs that the hospital has been providing in this area have been helpful and should be continued.

There are problems and questions remaining, however. Mooney believes that the therapists sometimes let themselves in for disappointment when they expect to accomplish too much. She notes that they are very enthusiastic and seem to take it out on themselves when every patient does not progress as far as they had hoped. Keeping up the morale of the therapists—and perhaps keeping their expectations within reasonable limits—is seen as a continuing need. She also wonders about the less obvious, more controversial dimensions of therapy. It is easy to see that things the therapists do are useful. This includes emotional support, companionship, and, in some cases, physical assistance such as ambulating the patient mentioned above. But is there something else?

> Healing, I have a very difficult time with that. I don't know that much about it, what it really involves. Being a nurse, I have a thing about medical healing rather than psychic, if that's the right word for it. I have a lot of questions about it right now, and so sometimes I might be very negative.

One of the most crucial positions in the hospital is that of head nurse on the intensive care unit. Dolly Gorman has had this responsibility for many years and has earned great respect from family as well as patients and staff. The therapy program did not take Gorman by surprise as much as it did most other staff members. She had read about "touch therapy" in the nursing literature and seen it portrayed on television, "so it wasn't so new to me."

> What I think is really interesting is that the patients do react to a one-to-one. They like having someone be with them. This is especially important when they are dying, just having someone holding their hands and being with them. I'm sure this helps a lot. As far as the healing goes — I don't know; it's a little of everything, treatments, and the therapy I think does help. We nurses, as much as we try to give them all the comfort we can, we don't have the time to stand there and hold their hand and talk to them for the longest while. We do our best anyway. I think it (the therapy) is helping. How much I don't know yet, because some of our patients can't tell us. But I know that the afternoon shift is very happy when the therapists come in because this is a bad time for patients. The sun goes down and they are fearful of night.

Gorman gave the example of a man who is up during the day in a wheelchair, pushing himself around, laughing, and interacting, but who suddenly becomes so short of breath in the evening that he has to have oxygen. "He's fearful of death during the night," Gorman observes. Lisa Hathaway sees this man in the evening and works to reduce his fears, a needed and valuable service.

Gorman shares in the general attitude that by far the most important consideration is the patient's condition, regardless of who does what to improve it. John Z. came up as an example with Gorman as well. She noted that actions on his behalf included Beverly's therapy, the religious faith and prayers of her staff, and excellent medical and nursing care. It is impossible to say precisely how much and in what ways each of these elements contributed to his recovery. "I think it was the combination of everything . . . including prayer and touching."

From her perspective, concerned with the care of some of the sickest and most debilitated patients in the hospital, Gorman sees the therapy program as valuable and the therapists themselves as "really committed. I think they love it. . . . They do it because they believe, and if there were more people like this, I think it would be fantastic." Nevertheless, she remains cautious about the long-term benefits of the program and about ways in which it might be refined.

"What I've seen I like, but I need to see more before I can make suggestions."

In summary, the program started at a time when nursing staff concern for adequate basic coverage made "something new and different" appear to be unwelcome. This initial problem perhaps could have been alleviated by more advance discussion. It is our impression, however, that the actual interactive experience was necessary before nursing staff would be in a position to make informed judgments. Having it to do over again, we would have tried to find some additional ways to introduce the program smoothly. We did feel limited in terms of what could be said to nursing and other clinical staff until we had seen the program in operation for ourselves. Certainly, those who introduce new therapeutic programs into geriatric facilities must take into account the problems and stresses of the moment and seek ways to reduce friction.

Staff acceptance of the program increased with familiarity. The therapists earned respect because of their dedication to the patients. The staff could see favorable results. Furthermore, many staff became interested in the therapeutic process, talking about it, reading, participating in seminars, and occasionally trying their own hand at it. Interpersonal difficulties became less frequent as referral and supervisory processes took refined shape, but at times there is still edginess about who deserves credit for what. There is by now a consensual view that one-to-one therapy of the type offered here makes a valuable addition to the efforts of other clinical services. Medical and nursing staff do not claim to know precisely what takes place in the therapeutic process. They have no trouble with the concept that a strong and positive personal relationship can help the patient make the most of his or her own resources and of what the hospital has to offer. About healing itself as an interpersonal (and, some would say, psychic) process, they are inclined toward cautiousness.

The one-to-one therapy program has demonstrated enough value to be accepted as part of the treatment spectrum. It has also attracted the interest of health care providers from other settings who would like to develop additional programs of this type. Such acceptance is encouraging. Nevertheless, it does not take the place of more precise types of evaluation which have now become more feasible because of the experience gained with the program.

FAITH, DOUBT, AND ERROR

Healers—whether thinking of themselves as physicians, priests, spiritualists, or whatever—have often brought the qualities of confidence and faith to their task. This much, at least, is clear from the historical perspective developed in Chapter 2. It has been observed that a strong intention to help, accompanied by belief in accomplishment, are "therapeutically active ingredients." As beneficial as this approach can be, however, it seems to invite error and snub the scientific approach. We cannot evaluate the relationship between faith, doubt, and error in therapeutic instances far removed from us in time and space, but it is possible to explore these dynamics within the confines of our own program. First it will be useful to touch briefly on faith and one of its neighbors—confidence—in a more general manner.

Therapists are not the only people who require a certain level of confidence. We all do. There may be a close relationship between the severity of the risks we face and the amount of confidence required to move ahead. Called upon to do something that is unusually difficult or that goes well beyond the information given, we are more likely to take up the challenge if we have a confidence that borders on faith. What we call *faith*, however, involves more than confidence in oneself. It assumes that the universe holds some power for the good and, furthermore, that the individual has access to this force, divinity, or principle. Looked at in this way, even the statistician acts on faith: the laws of chance are provided by a universe that obliges by being either so incredibly unorganized or so incredibly complex that randomness can serve as a fundamental concept. Every confident person must also have a certain degree of faith, no matter how disguised. Therapist, statistician, and every individual who moves beyond the known must assume a universe whose mode of operation supports one's own. It follows that either loss of confidence ("I am not capable") or loss of faith ("The universe destroys") inhibits wholehearted action.

These considerations are relevant to the technique as well as philosophy of therapy. Although we concentrate here on therapy with the aged, there is more general application as well. The Cushing Hospital therapists characteristically speak and act as though they have a kind of faith going for them. It is difficult to discuss faith in an even-minded way. Some people accept faith on faith, and there is nothing more to be said. Others would prefer to dispense with the concept altogether or, at the least, deny it admittance to the realm of therapy and sociobehavioral science. Preferences aside, faith is relevant in this context as phenomenological and social realities: therapists feel that they are supported by a strong faith, and somehow communicate this to the patients. Whether or not this faith is connected to anything (a loving god or laws as yet unverified by science) is another matter.

Somehow the confidence and faith of the therapist recruits the same orientation not only from patients but also from other staff, contributing to a more optimistic interpersonal milieu. Confidence and faith, mixed in any proportion, has functional value for therapists themselves. With a sense not only of personal confidence but also of collaboration from benign powers in the world, the therapist is more likely to accept and stay with the most difficult problems.

So much for what is obviously positive. Time now for the problems!

Humans err. Humans in the intensity and complexity of clinical situations are perhaps even more prone to error. Might not faith and confidence obstruct self-perception of error? Even "unfaithy" therapists can have difficulty in recognizing all the self-involving dynamics involved in their work. Defenses smoothly slide into place at times before even the most astute therapist can identify and deal with them. This would seem to be more than an ordinary hazard with therapists whose modus operandi owes much to faith.

Here is a kind of paradox, then: the faith that can move therapeutic mountains might also lead into unsuspected quicksand. The self-correcting process might be anesthetized by the headiness of faith. Put in a slightly different way, it is possible that healing efforts in which faith figures greatly produce their own variety of iatrogenic illness. The extreme is easy to recognize. The zealot flaming with a cause is correctly perceived as dangerous. Lacking perspective and balance, so secure in his or her beliefs that error and contradiction fail to register, the zealot is apt to do far more harm than good. The Cushing therapists are in no sense extremists. One must wonder, however, whether the faith and confidence necessary for their successful functioning exacts an *intrinsic* cost in error. In other words, we all make errors, but perhaps there is something in operating so much on faith that necessarily increases the probability.

The relationship of therapy to science is a controversial one. Some like to see therapy as the logical application of knowledge and principles that have been confirmed by empirical research. Others see therapy essentially as an interpersonal art form. Of most relevance here is the view that the therapeutic process itself should embody core principles of science. This is our own orientation. Research in the human sciences should be familiar to the therapist and utilized wherever possible. However, one is basically on one's own in the uniqueness of a particular therapeutic experience. Scientific generalities are of limited assistance here. What one can do, though, is to function in part as a scientist. This means remaining open to new observations, being not only willing but eager to revise one's ideas and actions based upon improved knowledge. This also strongly implies a critical, analytic approach. We are not referring to the psychoanalytic approach in particular, but to the process of taking a complex situation apart, getting to the specifics, looking beyond the obvious, allowing no assumptions to rest easily.

The listener found these concerns coming to mind as therapists presented case after case. He did not find much cause for concern about what the therapists were doing as particular individuals but, rather, about the more general question: can the critical, restless, self-correcting emphasis of the scientific therapist coexist with the global and largely undefined faith that seems to make this kind of healing effective? Must we choose one or the other?

This question is still open and should remain so until good observations in abundance have been made by a variety of researchers and clinicians. Nevertheless, a few glints from our experience are worth reflecting on.

Note that the therapists did not rely on "pure faith." They engaged in a number of specific activities that appear to have value: sensory enrichment, physical contact, relaxation exercises, and guided imagery, to mention some that have found frequent usage. It might be parsimonious to conclude that faith played its most substantial role in supporting the therapist's venture into situations so difficult that many others would have considered such an effort doomed to failure. Once in the situation, the therapist would continue to be sustained by what we call faith, but treatment efficacy would depend greatly on what was actually done. This view perhaps contains part of the truth, especially if it is not taken in too simple a form. One of the things the therapist would "do," for example, was to radiate the sense that life could once again be "okay," that what was good within the patient and what was good within the universe could be linked.

This aspect of faith is not especially problematic. It is the behavioral or the interpersonal facet, faith helping to bring out the best in both therapist and client. More problematic is the cognitive aspect: how the therapist is conceptualizing the situation and whether or not faith blinkers the capacity to doubt and revise.

The case of Matilda D. raises this question explicitly. The therapist here is a person who regards herself as a healer and for whom faith is a keystone of life. (While as a group, the therapists can be described as people for whom faith is important, there are appreciable individual differences as well.) The therapist formed an intimate and comforting relationship with this dying woman. Asked to review her objectives, she replied in part:

> I know that everything I do is healing. I don't have to question my actions because I know that they always are the right actions. I know that I was what Matilda needed in this situation. I knew that my words would be right for her, that my intentions were always to soothe her and to help her cope with her pain and, as the issue came up, eventually to cope with her own death.

This self-assessment includes two components: intentions and actions. The therapist obviously feels her intentions are entirely in the patient's interests. This is not a singular attitude: chances are that virtually all staff in all hospitals would characterize their intentions in the same way. There are at least two problems in relying on self-judged good intentions: (1) people differ in their ability to implement good intentions because of experiential, situational, and other factors; (2) the intentions may be more complex, ambivalent, and multilayered than what is apparent to the helping person. The good intentions and confidence in doing the right thing occur within a belief system that features the sense of efficacious contact with benign powers in the universe, that is, faith made operational. Is there risk in this orientation? Yes, we would say so. The greatest risk perhaps would be the assumption that good intention necessarily leads to wise action—the road to you-know-where is still being paved with such mental bricks. If a person truly persists in this assumption, then monitoring of one's actions, developing alternative approaches, and learning from experience in general would be inhibited. This would be counter not only to a scientist-clinician model but to any accepted guide to professional conduct.

The concern expressed here was also put directly to the therapist:

Skillful therapists of all schools ask questions of themselves. "Did I handle this situation right? Did I understand what was happening? Could I have done better?" But you—you are always right! How could you recognize it if you were wrong? How do you evaluate and improve? As you can see, I am importing a whole different frame of reference from the one you have been using, a more traditional, professional, and scientific frame of reference. Deal with it.

And the therapist did. She referred to the fact that this had been her first case at the hospital and her first interaction with a dying patient. She said, "I had no frame of reference." This example might hold a significant clue for the role of faith not only in therapy but in other challenging activities as well. New to the hospital and new to relating to a dying person, the therapist relied upon her existing frame of reference. Faith could not tell her what specific actions to take, but could enable her to proceed with a clear sense of mission, bolstered by her own empathy for people in distress: "I only knew that I cared and that I loved her. And I knew she was in need when she was in need—even if I didn't know what she was in need of. I felt she needed my simply being there and praying for all that is best and highest for Matilda. To come to her—at that point—maybe that was the best I could do."

The therapist did not feel totally confident from moment to moment in the relationship. She was afraid she might be doing particular things wrong, and she even apologized at times. Although charged with faith, she had not earned her own full confidence as a therapist in this situation. Andrea George was, in fact, monitoring her actions and attempting to suit them increasingly better to the purpose. She was learning.

The faith manifesto turns out not to be nearly as dogmatic as it might appear on the surface (in this and in other instances that have come to our attention at CH). Faith gives a general sense of guidance and a bedrock. It is that-which-one-does-not-question while moving ahead in difficult circumstances. The therapeutic plan and specific actions, however, remain open to examination, reflection, revision. The manifesto also is more likely to appear "hard line" when it is in response to a novel challenge. People for whom faith is a major organizing force tend to seek each other's company. Challenge from quite another framework may not come frequently. The strictly professional therapist likewise might be taken aback if given his or her first determined challenge by one who is rooted in a spiritualistic tradition. Such encounters can be bruising but useful for all concerned.

The faith, doubt, and error dynamics usually do not show up quite as clearly as in the instance that has just been discussed. Here are a few other examples from cases presented in this book.

Some therapists believe that faith plays a direct role in healing. This is certainly the case with Lisa Hathaway who comments during her presentation of Alfred B.:

> There were nights when I'd go in and feel really sensational—very trusting and secure and loving. I would just send that whole energy, and not just through the hands. It doesn't happen through your hands—well, sometimes it doesn, but it's through your whole body. You feel a rush. One rush after another. You can just feel it working. In working with Alfred it was like a circle: I felt a going to him and then I could feel it coming back. I was a really tight bond.

In some way this sounds like an especially dangerous view—not only does faith strengthen the therapist but it also works in real but mysterious ways to promote healing. Analysis of a passage such as the above does not eliminate the element of mystery, but does bring it into a frame of reference that requires fewer assumptions:

1. The therapist acknowledges a relationship between her own sense of being on a particular occasion and her therapeutic efficacy. This is a relevant and too often neglected dimension. (Furthermore, it suggests that faith, whatever this might "really" be, is to some extent a state-dependent phenomenon and worthy of further investigation in that light.)

2. A sense of organismic involvement with the patient is described: not just mental, not just verbal, but approaching and occasionally achieving total. But what language, what concept can be applied to gather together these inner events? The vocabulary of inner states is more familiar to poets than scientists. Terms such as healing energy might be accepted as accurate descriptions of what is experienced—words for something that is hard to put into words.

3. Whether or not a subjective (and real) state that is acceptably described as healing energies has validity in an external sense is a separate question. (And if we had the answer to that one, you would have read it by now!)

There is a kind of semantic vagueness at times, then, when it is difficult to find words to match the experience. Added to this is an easily corrected vagueness owed to habit. In reporting her work with Mary P., the same therapist said that the patient did not *want* to awaken, did not *want* to respond to stimulation.

"How do you know that?"
"I know that because I know her . . . I just felt. . . ."

At this point it would seem that unexamined intuition was being joined with faith to yield a global and uncritical view. Not so.

"Come on, Lisa." Did you have some clues to work with? Did she ever say anything to you about this? How did you form these impressions?

It took the therapist a moment to focus on this: her mind and feelings were occupied with significant aspects of the relationship, but with seemingly picky questions. Once she had done so, however, a clear observational base for what had seemed to be unbridled intuition came forth:

"At mealtime, that's a good example. She knew when mealtimes were. She could hear the banging and clanging of dishes and whatever, waking everybody up. 'Come on, let's eat!' is what the sounds would say, and sometimes the staff would say it in words. This is when she would curl up in a fetal position and put her hands under her neck so nobody could get her hands. Or she would cover her mouth, or she'd really just form more of a shell with her body. She did this at those particular times of the day rather than any other time, and it just seemed clear to me."

This seems a reasonable example of a type of communication that occurred more frequently at first, less frequently later. Not yet accustomed to describing observational specifics and relating these to interpretations and conclusions, the therapists would seem vague or intuitive. Quite often, the specifics were there, had been noted, and could be recalled. Intuition—by which is meant here conclusions arrived on the basis of minimal clues—does not completely vanish when therapists provide detailed accounts of their observational and inferential processes. We could not deny, even if we wanted to, that a process answering to the name of intuition exists and at times appears startlingly effective. However, true intuition (whatever that is) should not be confused with incomplete or global reportage.

Provisionally, it seems to us that a therapist can be inspired, encouraged, and in a sense, guided by faith and yet be a careful observer both eager and capable of learning through experience. Good observational (especially self-observational) skills require much attention and cultivation, with or without the presence of faith. Therapy with the old, sick, and helpless makes great demands on both head and heart. The most effective therapists will be those who value the intellectual and the emotional dimensions of their being and who are determined to continue their personal development even as they reach out to those in desperate circumstances.

REFERENCES

Birren, J.E., Butler, R.N., Greenhouse, S.W., Sokoloff, L., and Yarrow, M.R., (Eds.). *Human aging: A biological and behavioral study.* Bethesda, Md.: United States Public Health Service, 1963.

Kelly, G. *The psychology of personal constructs.* New York: W.W. Norton and Sons, Inc. 1955.

INDEX

Isolation
   and perceptual and cognitive dis-
      abilities, 183–184, 186, 190
   It's okay response, 75, 78–79, 82, 85,
      101, 103, 111, 113, 116, 130,
      144, 149, 173–174, 176, 178
   discussion of, 184–185, 212

Jealousy, 108–109, 177

Laying-on-of-hands, 9, 12, 19, 23,
   25–26, 196
Love, importance of, 25–27

Manic behavior, 145, 148
Massage, 11, 165–166, 168, 191–192
Medical science, 27–30, 47–49
Meditation, 116–117, 119, 133, 139
Memory loss, 87–88, 90, 105, 164
Mesmer, Anton, 14–16
Mesmerism, investigation of, 17–19
Mimic, 158, 175
Misdiagnosis, 17
Modern medicine, evaluation of
   negative aspects, 47–48
   positive aspects, 49–51
Multiple impairment, 3–4, 57
Music in therapy, 72–73, 102,
   112–115, 137
Mutual benefit from therapy, 73, 112,
   169

Negative thoughts
   effects on illness, 37–40
   of institutionalized, 58
   and recuperative functions, 49
Neurohypnotism, 19
Night terror, 72, 75–76, 171, 194,
   208
Nonverbal healing, 22–27
Nonverbal responses, 75, 80–82, 86,
   102, 153, 172, 186
Nonverbal suggestions, 44–45
Nursing shortage, 2, 61–62, 204, 206

Old (state of being), 197
One to one therapy, 65, 205–206, 209
Organic brain syndrome, 57

Paranoia, 71, 73, 145, 166
Perkins' "tractors," 45–46

"Pest house," 21
Philosophy, 72, 75, 81, 192–196
Philosophy of care, 4
Physician as servant of nature, 13
Placebo, 8, 10, 25
   effects, 46–47
Positive suggestions, 84, 101, 147,
   149, 189, 194–196
Praise, 89, 96, 102, 106–107, 113,
   141–142, 145–146, 158
   (see also Encouragement)
Pseudocyesis, 42
Psychic experience, 74, 153
Public facilities, 2

Relationships, 121–122, 179, 209
Relaxation, 84–85, 96–97, 137, 147,
   184, 188, 198, 212
Religious belief, 113–114, 145–146,
   174–175, 196

Sacred snakes, 11
Self-healing process, 9, 13, 30
Self-limiting illness, 12, 17
Self-suggestion, 20
Sensory enrichment, 75, 80, 102, 105,
   107, 212
Sickness, 197
Sleep, 20–21
Smiles, 72, 75, 80, 86, 93, 101, 106,
   114, 125, 159, 173, 178
Spiritual concerns, 113, 121, 195–196
Staff views of therapy
   and healing, 79, 98–99, 207
   need for basic care, 204–207
   negative feeling, 152, 160–162, 204,
      209
   no harmful effects, 202–203
   positive effects, 202, 209
Stress effects, 38–39
Sudden death, 40
Suffering, 194
Suggestion, 9–10, 13, 16, 20, 49, 183
Suggestive potency, 49
Suggestive therapy, 19, 22
   strengths and limitations, 43–47
Sulfonamides, 8, 28
Surgery, development of, 29
Sustagin, 159

Tardive dyskenesia, 193
Tarnkappe, 67

ABOUT THE AUTHORS

Robert Kastenbaum, Ph.D. has pioneered psychological therapies and research with the elderly and with the terminally ill. A past president of the Division of Adult Development and Aging of the American Psychological Association and of the American Association of Suicidology, he also serves as editor of *International Journal of Aging & Human Development*, and *Omega, Journal of Death and Dying*. He is now professor of gerontology at Arizona State University.

Theodore X. Barber, Ph.D. has been conducting psychological research for a quarter of a century. He is the author of more than 180 papers in professional journals and has written or edited seven books, including *Hypnosis, Imagination, and Human Potentialities* and *Pitfalls in Human Research*. He is continuing his clinical research as a staff member of Cushing Hospital.

Cheryl C. Wilson, Ph.D. has worked as a psychologist with the Sister Kenny Rehabilitation Hospital (Minneapolis) and as a postdoctoral research fellow in hypnosis and human potentialities at the Medfield (Massachusetts) Foundation. For the past three years she has been a researcher and therapy supervisor at Cushing Hospital.

ABOUT THE AUTHORS

Beverly Ryder graduated with honors in psychology from The University of Massachusetts–Boston and is presently senior therapist in the Cushing Hospital Supportive Services Department. She is also a speaker and consultant for the development of supportive therapy programs for geriatric patients.

Lisa Blair Hathaway is an artist and therapist who draws upon the healing tradition. In addition to her therapeutic work at Cushing Hospital, she teaches and counsels on meditation, care of the dying, and other topics and serves as a volunteer for Hospice at Home of Wayland (Mass.).

Date Due

JUN 7 1982		
MAR 8 9 '07		
JAN 29 '92		
OCT 05 '93		
OCT 19 '93		